scarred but smarter

A CANCER MEMOIR

NATALIE HOLLAND

Scarred but Smarter: A Cancer Memoir
Second Edition

ISBN-13: 978-1717473479

ISBN-10: 1717473474

Printed by CreateSpace, an Amazon.com Company

For the one who is my partner in crime,
the one who cheers me on and makes me laugh.
You remain my humble masterpiece, my David.

For my girls, you are my everything.

Table of Contents

Prologue

The Why

Prologue

What began as a catharsis for me evolved into so much more. In an effort to sort through the flurry of thoughts and emotions coursing through me, I put pen to paper in the fashion of a journal. While writing my thoughts began to extend well beyond just my personal experience and emotions. I wanted to know more about cancer, and I wanted to attempt finding answers to some questions. It sort of snowballed from there. The more I researched, the more I wanted to share my findings with others. However, I was a little reluctant to bite the bullet and approach the whole thing like a book as opposed to a diary.

My intention is to bring deeper awareness. With every story told, someone somewhere learns something new. I have learned, and continue to learn, each time someone shares a bit of their personal life story. With all that collective knowledge, it is my hope that we can unearth…some new answers…some better coping mechanisms…some improved treatments….some earlier detections…some sound prevention strategies….and a whole lot of hope.

Encouragement from others compelled me to just do it. There were two friends in particular who inspired me to take the plunge. One was my friend Crystal. During one of our chats, she shared the following with me:

"May the blessings released through your hands cause the windows to open in dark minds.
May the suffering your calling brings be but Winter before the Spring.
May the companionship of your doubt restore what your beliefs leave out.
May the secret hungers of your heart harvest from emptiness its sacred fruit.
May your solitude be a voyage into the wilderness and wonders of God.

May your words have the prophetic edge to enable the heart hear itself.
May the silence where your calling dwells foster your freedom in all you do and feel.
May you find words full of divine to find warmth to clothe the dying in the language of dawn.
May the slow light of Christ's Communion be a sure shelter around your future"
-David Walker

Around the same time another precious person by the name of Jeanne said to me: "If not you, who? If not now, when?". So, I took it as a sign to press forward. If the words in this book help even one person, then the hours I spent writing it will have been worth it. I know, I know...sounds so cheesy and cliche, right? But I mean it. I do! Now, if you expect this book to be eloquent and beautifully penned like the quote from David Walker, then this is NOT the book for you! Ha! I appreciate and adore elegantly written books, but in no way do I possess that kind of talent. And I should add now that I love Jesus, but I do curse on occasion. And I drink a little. (Have you seen the Ellen video where Gladys Hardy calls in? It's worth a Google!) If you are looking for an account from a real mom-wife-sister-daughter-friend and how she tangled with some cancer and came out better on the other side, then keep reading.

This book consists of two parts. The first is a walk through my personal experience with breast cancer. The second sheds some light on all the scary things lurking in our every day lives and tips on how to easily make substitutions for said scary things. You can (and I hope you will) read the book in its entirety, or you can read either half independently of the other. I thank you for reading this far, and hope you find some helpful things throughout the book.
XOXO
Natalie

One

Uh oh.

Never. At age 36, I really thought I had learned the lesson of "never say never", as time and again I'd said "Never This" and "Never That" only to be proven wrong and then some. As a young college student who'd aced high school with straight As, I thought I'd never ever fail a college course. Whooooops! It happened. I certainly did not enter into my first round of matrimony expecting divorce. Wrong, again. I never thought I would find endearing, lasting love with someone I met in a bar. Enter my husband, David. (So happy I was wrong about that particular "never"!) Apparently though, I have not yet mastered the lesson of "never say never" as I never, ever, ever considered that my "To Do" list would include fighting cancer…in my thirties…with two pre-teen daughters….a potty-training toddler….and a deployed husband. I can say that this is true of "never": I NEVER saw it coming.

Let me back up a month. Life was rocking along. My international-man-of-mystery husband David is often deployed. So after a decade of teaching high school science, I had recently resigned from my position to be a full time mom and to figure out what I wanted to do with myself next. After much thought, I had decided that I wanted to teach Pilates. It would be a nice fit for me. I had fallen in love with the method. This would allow me to continue teaching, but on a flexible schedule and to a different audience. Along with helping others restore themselves through physical movement, I could incorporate my B.S. in Nutrition and Dietetics into wellness protocols. It felt good to have a plan! I had just begun the Pilates certification process, and I was so excited to be moving in the right direction. Other things in my life seemed to finally be falling in place as well. We had recently sold a house which was a long holdover of the housing bubble burst, which came with a huge sigh of relief.

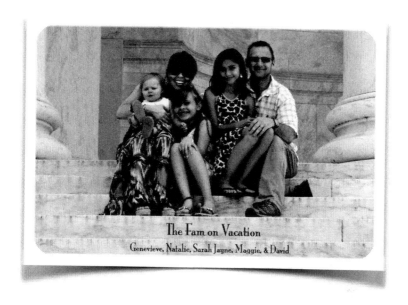

The Fam on Vacation
Genevieve, Natalie, Sarah Jayne, Maggie, & David

Like I said, life was moving along and things were falling into place. No sooner than the ink was dry on the housing contract and we had breathed that huge sigh of relief, I found it. I found a dayuuuum lump. I was literally scratching an itch. I had done plenty of self-exams in the past, but I must admit that it was not with absolute consistency. Still, I had done them enough to know that the lump felt new and foreign. I tried for a few days to ignore it, hoping it would sneak away as quietly and quickly as it had crept up. No such luck. Upon mentioning it to David, he insisted that I should have it checked.

I am typically a wait-and-see gal. For me, it usually seems to work best to chill and let things resolve themselves. I really loathe confrontation. I am, after all, the middle daughter - the peace-maker. But in this case, something compelled me to take action. I am sure the many breast cancer awareness campaigns I had been exposed to in the past helped push me in the right direction. But mostly, it was that quiet, guiding voice inside of me…women's intuition perhaps…that moved me forward. Divinely guided intuition, no doubt.

So, I made an appointment with my ob-gyn doctor. I figured it would be worth the peace of mind to hear that it was likely a cyst or something of the sort. After all, around 80%+ of all discovered lumps are benign. Plus, I was THIRTY SIX. No family history. Healthy weight. Exerciser. Had my babies relatively young. Breastfed them. Ate my veggies.

Clearly, it would be a cyst. Surely. Absolutely.

At least that is what I wanted to think.

Spurred by the data driven & science loving side of me, I continued to dig through more research. I completed some online breast cancer assessment tools. (There is a good one on cancer.gov.) The questionnaire was super easy. You select answers from drop-down menus and let the computer crunch away. My results: Lifetime risk of developing breast cancer by age 90: 11.3%. My five year risk of developing breast cancer: 0.3%. POINT THREE PERCENT. Less than one. Now I am thinking, "Y'all. I am golden. There is almost zero chance that this lump is cancer. Maybe I should cancel my appointment.".

Still, that little voice inside me said to go anyway.

While waiting the few weeks for my appointment to roll around, I am busy with kids and life in general. Maggie (12) has begun 7th grade. Sarah Jayne (10) has begun 5th grade. Genevieve (2) is home with me. David has crossed the pond to Afghanistan.

October 9 arrives, and it is time for my appointment. My doctor checks the lump. Though she agrees that I am young with little risk for breast cancer, she said the feel of the lump warrants a mammogram...hopefully to rule cancer out. No problem! Again, the peace of mind from the imaging will be worth it.

I call to schedule my mammogram. There is almost immediate availability, but Sarah Jayne's 11th birthday is in just a few days time. I want the appointment to fall *after* her birthday on the super-far-fetched-off-chance that the news is no bueno.

October 24 is the date I am given.

In the weeks that follow, as I wait for my appointment, I often find myself praying for strength. Even though I hope the lump is nothing, and even though I know my risk for malign results is tiny, I notice that my prayers are not pleading that the lump is nothing. Rather, I find myself asking for guidance, for strength, and for peace. Maybe something very deep inside of me knows that something isn't right. Again, I think it is that divine guiding voice trying to prepare me for what is to come.

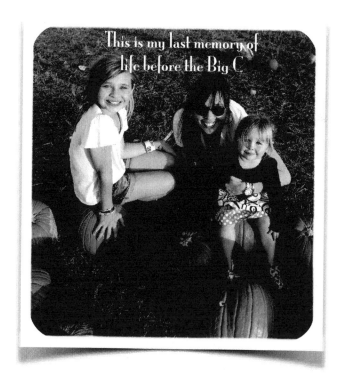

This is my last memory of life before the Big C

October twenty-fourth arrives. My appointment is in the morning. Since I have the luxury of a babysitter for most of the day, I have big plans. Mammogram….lunch with a friend…Pilates training. I love a full, productive day! I arrive at the imaging suite which is a breast-specific center. They do all boobs all day long, so I assume they are very good at what they do. I sign in and begin filling out my paperwork. I am the youngest woman in the waiting room. (I suppose that was a portent of future events, as I would often find myself in the situation of being the youngest.) My name is called; I change into a gown and wait. I nervously wait. There are many magazines to read to pass the time. Since it is October, every single one is full of articles about breast cancer. Every. Single. One.

Wait, wait, wait, wait. My heart is beating a little too fast, and my tummy has butterflies. Finally, my name is called. The technician is very personable and sweet, and for this, I am thankful. She proceeds with the mammogram, starting with the right breast. Smassssshhhhhhh then smooooosh a little more. Who knew a boob could literally be turned into a pancake?!?! Geez. I am instructed to take a deep breath and remain very still as the image is taken. Ok- now breathe. Time to repeat the process for the left. I slip back into my gown and return to the waiting area. I flip through more magazines, half reading and half just zoning out. Some time later, the technician returns and lets me know that radiologist would like to add an ultrasound. Uh-oh. I knew that meant something was at least suspicious. Surely the ultrasound would confirm a cyst of some sort, right? Yes, yes….the ultrasound will be to confirm a cyst.

It was in the dimly lit ultrasound room that I began to suspect that my worst fear may be realized. As the ultrasound technician was imaging the suspicious area, I proceeded to make small talk…nervous chatter really. I don't remember any of the conversation except the part where I mentioned that ultrasounds were so much more fun when looking at a wiggly baby. She said nothing. Crickets. I supplied a bit of nervous laughter. The tech chimed in with silence and a small, pity-laced smile. A big hint that something was really amiss. Damn.

I return to the waiting room. Unsure of how much time passes, I read even more breast cancer articles in the October glossies. Finally, the original technician lets me know that the radiologist would like to see me to discuss my images. Breathe in. Breathe out. I can do this. I enter a softly-lit office where I am introduced to the doctor. Images of my breasts are visible on the screens behind her. She is very polite and kind, but she gets right to business by directing my attention to a particular area of interest on one of the images. "You see this," she says. "It has all the hallmarks of a cancerous tumor."

In that instant, it is as if everything has been sucked out of the room. The air is gone. Sound is gone. People disappear. I am left with the feeling that I am clearly having a nightmare and will wake at any moment covered in sweat, heart racing but grateful that it was only a bad dream. The moment is simultaneously eternal and brief. CANCER. She thinks I have *CANCER*. I know that my life has just changed forever. From this point on, time will be marked by that sense of before and after. Hold up...she is still talking. Snap out of it. Breathe and focus, Natalie. Breathe in. Breathe out. Pay attention. Okay, she is talking again about the image on the screen. Yes, I see the little monster on the monitor. Yes, it looks like all the images I researched before my appointment. Yes, I understand why she finds it suspicious. Yes, I see why she thinks it is cancer. But why is she telling ME all of this? Because I know that cannot be my breast we are talking about. Simply can't. I cannot have cancer. Once again, I need to snap back to reality, since the doctor is still speaking. She is speaking, but I am not quite comprehending the words. My mind is already racing with a million and one questions. I think my mouth is even hanging open. Agape, perhaps wishing I could eat the answers right from the air.

I hear her say, "Is anyone with you today?". I tell her that I am alone. "I would like to biopsy both breasts today if it is possible for you to return after lunch." My thoughts are so fuzzy, but I manage to tell her that I need to call my babysitter as my husband is in Afghanistan. My older kids are in school, and the youngest is with the babysitter. I send a message to my sitter, Louisa…Saint Louisa, and she has no problem staying, so I let the doctor know that I can return.

In a daze, I wander down the hall to the dressing room. I am wracking my brain for the best way to tell my husband via FaceTime that I probably have cancer. Is there an eloquent way to break the news of cancer? Is there a way to do it that spares some of the pain? As soon as I get in my car, I ring him up. All hope for eloquence is lost for as soon as I see him, the only thing I could blurt through tears is, "She thinks I have cancer.". Honestly, I do not even remember what words he used, but they made me feel better. He assured me that no matter what, we would tackle it together. *Thank you, Lord, for sending me a mate who can quell me from 6000 miles away.* I am a lucky girl.

The next hour or so passes in a total blur. I call my parents. October 24 happens to be their anniversary. Again, I search for the right words. It pains me to think of breaking the news to them. Once again, articulateness fails and the words tumble out something like this, "Mom, Dad…Happy Anniversary. Um, I think I have cancer.". And again, I do not remember exactly what they said, only that they reassured me that it would all be alright. And that they would book a flight and zip right out to San Antonio. Evermore, I am reminded of how blessed I am.

I call a few girlfriends, and then it is time to return to the imaging center. First order of business: a core needle biopsy for my right breast. This is an ultrasound-guided biopsy. First, the area is numbed with a local anesthetic. The, a large hollow needle is inserted and it "punches" out cores of tissue samples. The process is repeated until the doctor gathers as much tissue as needed, usually three to six times. It feels uncomfortable, but the pain is very manageable. However, the accompanying noise is unnerving…like a loud, automatic hole puncher. Second order of business: stereotactic core needle biopsy for my left breast. This is used when suspicious micro calcifications are revealed on the mammogram but are not palpable or seen on the ultrasound. X-ray equipment is used for imaging. For this, I have to lie face down on an exam table with my left breast dangling in a hole. (Dooooo your boobs hang low, do they wobble to and fro, can you…..I can't help it. The song popped into my head.) The breast is then compressed VERY tightly, and a needle is inserted to take samples.

By this time I am mentally and physically spent. My mind has reached its limit, and it is momentarily almost blank. Dazed. Confused. Worried. I do not even know where my thought process should be at this point. So overwhelmed. I am aware that tears are slowly and silently streaming down my face. I am not hysterical or sobbing, but I can't seem to stop the flow of tears. I am positioned so that I cannot move my arms to wipe them away. The sweet, kind nurse by my side during the exam gently wipes them for me. I am thankful for her compassionate thoughtfulness.

Since that whirlwind day, many have asked me if I thought the radiologist did the right thing by telling me I likely had cancer before she had access to any pathology reports. My answer: undoubtedly. She is the radiologist in a breast-imaging center. She looks at boobs all day every day. Young boobs. Old boobs. Big boobs. Small boobs. Healthy boobs. Sick boobs. I would most definitely consider her a boob expert. Because she cut right to the chase and shared her thoughts with me, I was able to ask her many questions (once I gathered my wits, of course). "When can I expect results?". "Who will call me with the news? Or do I call someone?". "If cancer is confirmed, what in the world do I do next?". She was able to answer the questions I was coherent enough to ask at the time. I thought she was wonderful. What often takes two weeks or more…mammogram, ultrasound, biopsy…took one day for me. One. She also gave me her card and told me to call her personally if I had not heard from my doctor by the close of business on Friday. Answers that take weeks for some were going to be given to me in less than 48 hours.

After a grueling day, it is time to go home, relieve the babysitter, and put on my best happy-mom face. I arrive home and call David once more from the driveway. I need a pep-talk before returning to my "normal life" waiting inside. By now, it is about two in the morning where he is, yet he has remained awake until the wee hours to be instantly available to me as I finish trudging through this scary day. Though worlds away, his love and support are undeniable. He proceeds to tell me an extremely funny story about something that had happened a few days earlier. Now…I can't share the story, because he would surely divorce me, but the point is that he sat on it for two whole days knowing that I just might need a good laugh on October 24, 2012. It made me guffaw! He knew exactly how to cheer me up enough to be able to go inside our home and manage being both mom and dad, homework helper, diaper changer, dinner maker, bath giver and book reader for the remainder of the day. One of my favorite things to do is laugh, and David always knows how to crack me up. Again, I am thanking my lucky stars because laughter can soften some of life's hardest blows. I'd be one step away from a nervous breakdown without some comic relief.

I head inside and relieve Louisa. I take care of all the afternoon and evening mom duties with the girls. After I tuck the girls in their beds and the house grows quiet, my soul feels as heavy and dark as the night outside. I know that over the horizon, the sky is bright…not because the sun has risen, but because my David is there. I am soothed knowing that I am blessed with an amazing partner to help see me through the ups and downs of life.

The next day, Thursday, passes in a total blur. My sweet girlfriend, Heather, brings flowers and coffee. She helps me make a Target run since I am not supposed to lift much. (I was sore and bruised from the biopsies, and one site had already developed a giant hematoma. The first of many bumps and bruises.)

Friday arrives, and so do my parents. My parents have never been big on displays of affection…not in the traditional sense anyway. They are not big huggers or big smoochers. Talking about emotions makes them uncomfortable. Anything mushy makes them squirm. If you ever watched That 70's Show, you can picture my dad as Red. My mom was more like Mama from "Mama's Family"…only with the style, panache, and laughter of Lucy of "I Love Lucy". Though they are never really forthcoming with the "I love yous", their support my entire life has been as ubiquitous as the sun. If there was a program at school, they were there. Sporting events…check! They were there. Kickball and homemade ice cream in the neighborhood…right in the middle. Big life events like college graduation, the birth of my first child, the collapse of my first marriage….there they were. When I called with the news that I probably had cancer, without hesitation, they hopped on a plane.

The day passes and we busy ourselves with errands and kid stuff, all while willing the phone to ring. Finallllllly, I call my doctor just before five. She is still at her office, and my pathology report has just come across her desk. She keeps me on the phone as she gives it a look, and then she confirms the suspected: I have cancer.

Cancer. Cancer. Cancer.

Such a succinct word with an enormous and far-reaching impact. With that one word, I know my life has forever changed in a multitude of ways.

Now it was time for the run through the gauntlet to begin. I have decided that the cancer road is more like a gauntlet than a marathon. It is long and grueling like a marathon, but it has so many tricky and unexpected challenges with no clear finish line.

Though the diagnosis confirmed cancer, the whole situation still felt surreal. Me? Cancer? No way. I still couldn't even say "I have cancer". It would take a long time before I could actually speak the words aloud. I needed a game plan. I always feel better with a plan. Where was I supposed to start, though? I wish I'd had a "Field Guide for Cancer". I was anxious for a plan, but I was clueless about where to begin. Who do I call? Who will be on my care team? What comes next? Luckily, I have a friend who is an oncology nurse. Carole was able to guide me through the process and point me in the right direction. Again, thank God for friends! At this point, I am beginning to see that it takes a village to help a cancer sister out.

I was able to get an appointment for the very next week with a highly regarded oncologist. Though a week was very quick, the wait felt like an eternity. This cancer gig is a lot like the army life...so much "hurry up and wait". The appointment is scheduled for Halloween Day, which is also my mom's birthday. "Happy Anniversary, mom and dad. I have cancer. Happy Birthday, mom. Let's party at the cancer center!"

The appointment day arrives, and my mom and I meet my doctor. We dial David in via FaceTime. (It is a great millennium to be alive! I love modern technology.) I immediately like my doctor. He is warm and conversation flows easily. He has a sense of humor, explains things well, and I get the sense that he is well-schooled on current research. I will go ahead and throw this in now....it is so important to LIKE YOUR DOCTOR. Not all doctors are created equally. Some are phenomenal. Some are duds. Some are somewhere in the middle. In the case of an oncologist, you will have a long-term relationship together, and you will be making life and death decisions with this person. If you don't get a warm and fuzzy from your doctor, nix him! (Or her!) There's a sea of doctors out there. Find the one who is a good fit for you and your situation.

We spend time talking about my pathology report. The size of my tumor stages me at two. Because of the size, if my lymph nodes are negative, I will be Stage 2A...if they are positive, I will be stage 2B. Nodal status will be determined at the time of surgery. I am ER/PR +. Estrogen and Progesterone positive. This means that both estrogen and progesterone feed my tumor. My measure of positivity is extremely high for both hormones, which means that my cancer is FUELED by them. I am HER2 negative. Human Epidermal Growth Factor Receptor 2. HER2 positive cancers tend to grow faster, but there are medicines specifically for HER2 positive breast cancers. I have a very high Ki67 score, which is a bit worrisome. A high Ki67 score suggests a faster-growing, more aggressive cancer, rather than a slower, "laid back" one. (Aaand does anyone else feel that "laid back" and "cancer" should never be spoken in the same sentence?)

I am furiously taking notes the whole time. I know there are things I will want to research. I also know there are parts of the conversation that seem clear now but will be all fuzzy later. Based on my age, the pathology report, and the aggressiveness of my tumor, my doctor recommends a bilateral mastectomy, chemotherapy, and hormone (well, anti-hormone…more on that later) therapy. So much to digest. It is a relief to know the plan. In the same breath, it is overwhelming.

Holy shit, the treatment road is going to be long.

Next up: lab work. My doctor will run more tests including a genetic panel. He is almost certain that I will test positive for BRCA1 or BRCA2 since breast cancer for a young, otherwise healthy woman with no family history is extremely rare. Off to the lab I go. I already have a hate/hate relationship with needles. Aaaarrrrggghhhh! Shots, no problem. Digging around for a vein….for the love! Makes me woozy. Thankfully, though the lab tech does not have a sparkling personality, she is a great sticker. At this point, sticking skills trump personality preferences. I donate enough blood to sate a vampire, then I head downstairs to meet with an oncology surgeon. I did not get the impression that he was my oncologist's first choice, but rather a suggestion prompted by insurance company. Apparently Tri-Care is not accepted by everyone.

My first impression is this: Come Hell or high water, I do not want this man operating on me! His nurse is blunt and rude. He rolls in looking like a disheveled Gene Wilder (I love me some Gene Wilder…but I wouldn't want him operating on me); sneezes; then extends his hand for a handshake. Ummmm yeahhhh, I totally want this man's hands all over me in the operating room….not. We discuss things for a few minutes. I ask about the possibility of a nipple sparing mastectomy, which David and I have already thoroughly researched. Though it is a newer approach, if all the specs are met which make someone a good candidate for the the procedure, it is just as safe as removing the nipples completely. It is as if he doesn't even hear me when I ask about this. He immediately answers no…with a wave of his hand…like someone swatting a fly…and moves on. Totally dismissive. I am completely annoyed that he would wave my question away like he was shooing a pest. I leave not really knowing what to think, and feeling trapped by my insurance options.

At any rate, it is time to head home…relieve the babysitter…do the school pick-up…celebrate my mom's birthday….and go Trick-or-Treating.

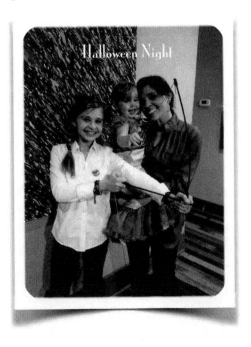

I still haven't shared the news with my girls. I was waiting until I met with my oncologist and had a better understanding of my diagnosis. Since I do not care to ruin Halloween, I decide the news can wait one more day. Bring on the chocolate.

Two

Making Plans

Suzanne. That is my middle name, but maybe it should have been "Procrastination". Or perhaps "HatesConfrontation". Natalie ProcrastinationHatesConfrontation Davis Holland. The meeting with my oncologist had taken place, so I could no longer delay sharing the news with my kids.

David was still overseas. Since Maggie was at her mother's house, he handled telling her to spare me from having to go through the process twice. Genevieve was only two at the time. She would not really understand the word "cancer". Though I would tell her at some point that "Mommy is sick" or that "Mommy has to have some booboos fixed", the big C word would not leave the same immediate impression on her as it would the older girls. That left Sarah Jayne to tell.

Over the week, I had taken time to read all those little pamphlets with advice on just how to go about sharing news like "I have cancer" with your child. She was barely eleven. I wanted so badly to be able to spare her any pain or worry. But really....how do you take the sting out of "cancer"? I approached it as honestly as I could. She knew that I'd had a few recent doctor appointments. I sat her down and reminded her of those appointments. I explained that my doctors had run some tests. Once again, the words tumbled out in a way that was far from polished or pain-free. I simply said that the tests had revealed that I have cancer.

There are no words for the way the look on her face made me feel. It told me she felt a mix of fear, bewilderment, shock, and sadness. Every single emotion a parent wants to spare their child was written all over her face and in her body language. Though I knew it was not my fault that I had cancer, I still felt completely responsible and incredibly guilty for evoking those emotions in her. Her first question....through tears.... "Mom, are you going to die?". Sigh.

My heart breaks into one thousand and one pieces.

That is a question I never thought I would have to answer for my young and tender hearted daughter. Tears fell…for the both of us. I spent some time answering more of her questions. "What is next? Will I get cancer, too?" So many questions. So many things that I was wondering myself. So many things that frightened me.

"Do not be afraid, for I am with you. Do not be discouraged, for I am your God. I will strengthen and help you. I will hold you up with my victorious right hand."
Isaiah 41:10

Comfort.

November third brings my PET scan…a first for me. I was remotely familiar with PET scans, but I had to refresh my memory about exactly how they identified tumors in the body. Here is my best layman's explanation. You begin by fasting. When you arrive for the exam, the first thing is a finger prick to check your blood sugar level. If all is well with the number, an IV is started and you are injected with a radioactive solution that will circulate in your body for an hour before the actual scan. For the scan, you are placed in a machine much like an open MRI machine. It takes about twenty minutes. The radioactive markers are attached to sugar molecules, which allows the metabolism of the sugar by the body to be seen on the scan. Tumors are hungry little devils since they are rapidly dividing. Ergo they metabolize sugar at a very high rate. In a healthy body, one would expect to see the radioactive sugar molecules being metabolized at an even rate throughout the body. If one area "lights up" with an unlikely concentration of sugar, this is indicative of a potential problem… possibly a tumor.

At this point, I am praying, "Please don't let me be a Christmas tree! For the love, do not let my body look like Clark Griswold got a hold of it." Oh, and "No whammies, no whammies, no whammies....STOP at that breast tumor!" (If you never watched the gameshow Press Your Luck, that last analogy may be lost on you.) The actual scan is not bad. After the injected solution circulates for an hour, I just have to lie still as the machine makes all sorts of noises. I actually drift to sleep for a bit. The IV wasn't bad, and the time in the machine wasn't either. However, it was tough to go home and not be able to hug my kids. Enough time has to pass so that the radioactive material is broken down and excreted from my body. The hardest thing about the test is waiting for my results. They arrive a week later, and thankfully, the only thing that lit up was my breast tumor. No surprise METS (metastases) were found. Hooooray!

The remainder of November consists of a lot of "hurry up and wait". Who hasn't prayed for patience? I know that I have. Well, ask and ye shall receive. I was now being given the trials to develop that patience. I will be the first to admit that being a patient patient is a CHALLENGE.

By this time, I knew that I was happy with my oncologist. He would be overseeing my master plan: chemo, hormone treatment, etc. However, I still had no idea what surgeon was going to perform my bilateral mastectomy, because it sure wasn't going to be disheveled Gene Wilder. Neither did I know who was going to reconstruct my boobs. I had been told by many that there was only ONE plastic surgery group in San Antonio to consider for reconstruction, because that was their specialty. Not augmentation. Not lifts. Not lipo. Not nose-jobs. Breast reconstruction. They were the specialists to use when one needed hooters built from scratch. It was comforting to know that I would be in great hands. Imagine my disappointment when I called to find out that they did not accept my insurance. I felt crushed and completely unsure of what to do next.

Attempting to move past the letdown, I started calling other local plastic surgery groups who accepted TriCare (my insurance). I found a handful who *did perform* reconstructive surgery, but they did not specialize in it. My research at this point had already helped me to understand that breast reconstruction and breast augmentation were two very different animals. I would be getting new boobs. From scratch. It would be a multi-step, multi-surgery process. (To this day is still bothers me when people say something to the tune of this…."Oh, too bad you had breast cancer, but at least you got a free boob job." I know they mean well, but when anyone says something like this, all I can think is that they have no idea what breast reconstruction involves. It is most def not a boob job. It is a rebuilding process after breasts have been amputated.) As I called around town, I got the same feeling from each office I contacted. I felt confident that any of the offices I called could do a great augmentation or facelift, but I did not find one office which made me feel as if they could handle a reconstruction with which I would feel satisfied. After many tearful conversations with David, he urged me to call the original office of choice and inquire about paying for the surgery out-of-pocket. He said that we would figure out a way to make it work.

I make the call. I get a quote. I almost choke!!!!! The quote comes in at FIFTY TO SIXTY THOUSAND DOLLARS….MINIMUM! And that 50-60k would need to be paid up front. Do I laugh? Do I cry? Though I have a good sense of humor about most things, I must admit that I cried about this setback. I can laugh about it now, but I found absolutely nothing funny at all at the time!

I feel deflated and at a loss for what to do next. I have a cancerous tumor growing inside of me. I want it out. Now. In fact, having it out yesterday would be even dandier.

By this time, my family already knew of my diagnosis. I decided it was time to come out of the cancer closet to the virtual world via social media. In poured an overwhelming amount of love and support. It made me decide that I would be as open as I could bear with my cancer journey. I wanted to shed light on what it is really like to have cancer. I wanted to raise awareness as much as possible. And honestly, all of the incredibly kind words of concern…all of the support…all of the prayers….it all pushed me forward. Especially the funny prayers. Y'all will hear me mention my friend Jeanne several times, because she is always saying some really funny shiz. Prime example:

Jeanne
Praying my good straight up prayers that God is holding your boobies in the palm of his hands and you feel some comfort. Love you, Nat! Fight like a girl. Bubbies ;) Lol. Maybe imagine that. I just imagined you looking at him holding your boobies... You were like What Up Lord ;) Hahahaha.
                   But bet you felt better
Me
Now I have this in my head...to the tune of "He's Got the Whole World in His Hands": He's got my whole boob in his hands, he's got my whole boob in his hands.....he's got the one with the cancer in his hands...he's got my boob and her sister in his hands..." I could go on and on. It's STUCK in my head now! But it is making me laugh- so thanks!!

Jeanne
I love you;) He does have your boobs in his hands;)

    I really hope no one reading finds that sacrilege…totally not meant in that way….a girl has gotta laugh.
    It was at this time that prayers for me began abounding. Concurrently, I saw them being answered. The very next day, a solution to my surgery conundrum presented itself. My oncology nurse friend asked me why I had not considered MD Anderson in Houston. I told her that the thought had crossed my mind, but that between pre-op, post-op, and expansion visits plus oncology and chemo treatment visits, there was no way I could handle it since it

was a three hour drive from San Antonio. She explained that I could do all of my surgical stuff there while keeping my oncologist in San Antonio. Oh. Well. Duh! Never occurred to me. See....I told y'all I needed a "Cancer for Dummies" book.

Prayers answered.

I was able to get an appointment with a surgeon she knew personally. Yasssssss! The appointment, however, was about three weeks away. On the surface, three weeks seems pretty zippy. When you know there is cancer growing inside of your body, zippy stretches into a lifetime. This did give me much time to think and prepare, though. It also gave David time to get home from Afghanistan.

As I waited for the surgery to take place and for treatment to begin, I had much time to think. Time to think is a good thing....except when it isn't. An idle mind is the devil's workshop they say. During that time, I had a gripping fear that cancer would take my life. I spent much of November imagining worst case scenarios. Fear of the unknown had a strong hold on me. I would think of my husband without his wife, my girls without their mother, my parents without their daughter, and my siblings without their sister. Imagining such scenarios broke my heart into a million pieces. Knowing what I am supposed to do with my life professionally has always shifted. Life circumstances and the acquisition of new knowledge tends to shape what we want to do with ourselves. However, one thing about which I have always been certain is that I always wanted to be a mother. I knew that my most important job would always be "Mom". The fact that the honor and joy of being a good mama may be cut short was terrifying. The fear was unlike anything I'd ever experienced. It would stop me in my tracks...cause my palms to go sweaty...my heart to race...and it would make me feel generally panicked. When that happened, I would literally take a deep breath and say a prayer. Breathe in. Breathe out. After enough breathing and praying, that peace which passes all understanding would wash over me, and I knew my prayers were being heard. I would pray, "Please don't let me die. Please. I can muster the strength for treatment. I can endure physical and emotional pain. I can learn to manage the fear of the unknown. But please, oh please don't let me die". I know that the faith of life everlasting is supposed to make us at peace with meeting our Maker...and it does...but I would be a liar liar pants on fire if I said that I was ready to leave this Earth and my family now. So I gave myself a Texas-sized attitude adjustment. I decided that live or die...cancer was not winning. If I let cancer change the very essence of my being, then it wins.

I am not letting it win.

It was during the same time that I thought often about the word "survivor". I decided then and there that survivorship should not be defined by how long you survive, but *how* you survive. It should be given meaning by the decision to take control of your life and LIVE. It is about doing everything in your power to survive cancer and to thrive during and after treatment. For me, careful attention to diet, exercise, attitude, and what I put on my body (shampoos, lotions, makeup, etc) helped give me a sense of control. It quells me knowing that I am doing all that I can to give myself the best chance for good health. I know that you can do everything right and still get cancer or have a recurrence, but living healthily goes a long way in reducing one's risk.

Survivorship is about living life to the fullest. None of us are promised tomorrow, but we are given free will to make the best decisions we know how. If any thought is stopping you from achieving your hopes and dreams, cast fear aside...throw caution to the wind...and get out there and make it happen....because life without risk is no adventure...and that is a shame! I think I will live until I die, thank you very much.

Also during this time, people started to use "Fight like a girl!" to encourage me. You guessed it...this got me to pondering as well. I guess the phrase means different things to different people. For me it means many things. It is about determination. Strength. Defiance. It is about making a commitment to stand up to cancer and to anything or anyone standing in the way of your dreams. It is about not giving up in the face of adversity. It means for YOU to claim YOUR POWER. It means for you to dig deep and find what motivates you. It means to educate yourself, for knowledge is power. Fighting like a girl also encompasses allowing others to help you. You are not an island. Let others lend you strength when you need it. Draw on that strength by allowing others to physically and emotionally support you. This can be especially challenging if you are accustomed to being independent to a downright stubborn degree. But do it. Let others in. You will be glad you did. Girls are made of much tougher stuff than sugar and spice. Breathe in. Breathe out. Stand tall. Take Control. There is no time like the present to realize that if anything is keeping you from living a happy and fulfilling life, you can overcome it. Prevail. Empower yourself. Persevere. Kick ass. Fight like a girl.

So now we are in the middle of November, and my David makes it home from Afghanistan. He will be able to make my rounds of initial appointments at MD Anderson. I am always elated when he arrives home. No matter how many times we are separated by deployments, homecomings never get old. Never! When he is home...the complex stuff seems easier...life seems lighter...laughter abounds.

David is home one day and we head to Houston the next. Saint Louisa is taking care of the girls. We arrive late and spend the night in the hotel attached to M.D. Anderson Cancer Center (MDA). Early the next morning, we are looking out the window before my day of appointments begins, and David coins it "Cancer Mecca", which really made me laugh. The place is HUGE and encompasses several city blocks.

The day begins with registration. Next comes imaging: mammograms and ultrasounds. At least this time I already know that I have cancer which takes some of the anxiety away. At MDA, they like to image you realllllllllly well. I change into my robe and wait for my technician. (Yes, a posh robe. Nice robes beat crusty hospital gowns any day!) I lose count of how many times I am mammogrammed. It is so many times that I think I may not need a bilateral

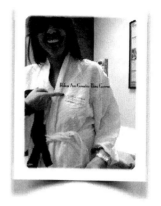

mastectomy after all because I am certain that my boobs are about to be squeezed right off my chest. Thankfully, I have an extremely sweet and personable tech....makes all the difference! Mammograms are followed by ultrasounds. Thankfully, no new tumors are found.

The next day we meet with my surgeon, and I immediately like him. He is very open to a two-way conversation....talking *with* me instead of *to* me. We talk about the possibility of a skin and nipple sparing bilateral mastectomy. Based on my imaging, he tells me that it is a very likely possibility, but that the only way to know for sure is to see exactly where the tumor is located during surgery. It will have to be an acceptable distance from the skin. I let him know that I was comfortable with him making that decision during surgery, which meant that I would not know which approach was used until I woke from surgery. If this approach is used, every morsel of my breast tissue will be removed, but my skin will remain. No matter whether or not the nipples would be saved, expanders will be placed in my chest wall after the breast tissue is removed. This involves making an incision in the top layer of the pectoralis major muscle, peeling it back, placing the expander behind the chest wall, then using a mesh material to stitch muscle back to muscle thus making a sling for the expander. Eventually, muscle grows through the mesh material. The expanders are filled with saline and have metal ports which can be accessed by a needle. The expansion process will take place over several months, and my plastic surgeon will oversee the process. It is explained to me that since I will be missing all of my breast tissue, that I will never have the sensation of breasts again. With or without my nipples, the best-case-scenario for my skin is that I will regain "protective sensation". I ask my surgeon to explain exactly what he means by that. He says, "You know, like to avoid burning yourself when you are cooking and such." To which I laughed and said, "Oh yes, since I spend so much time naked in the kitchen, especially with pre-teens and toddlers whirling around me." So he proceeds to explain that he's had patients burn themselves through their clothing from the steam of boiling water. Awesome! Not only do I have to worry about not burning down the house because I forgot to turn off the oven, but now I have to worry about singeing my foobs. Annnndddd he had a patient who severely burned herself while leaning against her hot car in the summer. I picture my skin melting....YIKES! The thought is pretty horrifying to me. South Texas Summer heat....the struggle is real, y'all! Ok- I digress.... Also during the surgery, I will undergo an sentinel node biopsy. My axillary lymph nodes on the right side (the cancerous side) will be dyed and some of them removed. The breast is first injected with a dye, and the nodes in the axillary region that first pick up that dye are the sentinel nodes. They will be removed during surgery and tested for cancer. If they are free of cancer, one can assume that the remaining nodes in the region are cancer-free as well. If they have cancer, then a decision has to be made about whether to remove all of the axillary nodes or not. (Why not just remove all of them at any rate? Any time nodes are removed, one is at risk for lymphedema....for the rest of their life. Lymphedema involves swelling....usually of the affected arm and hand, though it can be anywhere. The swelling can be from mild to severe. The more nodes that are removed, the greater the chance of experiencing lymphedema.) The prediction is that the surgery will last around seven hours. It will begin with the oncology surgery team followed by the plastic surgery team.

Some may wonder why I chose mastectomy over lumpectomy and a bilateral mastectomy at that. I was not a candidate for lumpectomy as imaging at MDA revealed multiple cancerous focal points extending toward my chest wall. So much tissue would have to be removed to get clear margins that there wouldn't be enough tissue remaining to make up a breast. Research shows that the mortality rate is roughly the same for mastectomy and lumpectomy, but that lumpectomy does have a bit higher rate of recurrence. I knew that removing both breasts did not ensure that my cancer would never return. However, it felt like the right decision for me. My reasoning was that since there was a perfect storm that allowed cancer to grow in one breast, then what would be keeping it from setting up house in the other one. Additionally, breast cancer in young women (diagnosed under 40) is more likely to return. So many times people have said to me, "You are young and otherwise healthy. That is a good thing as far as cancer is concerned. You will be able to kick it and never have it return.". What they do not realize is that a vast body of research shows that being young with breast cancer is an independent predictor of adverse outcome. For some reason, tumors are more aggressive…they tend to recur more often….and they kill more often. Sooooooo, I wanted both breasts gone. Vamoose, boobies. (And yes, I know that cancer can return even with no breasts.) Of course, anyone in the same situation should do their own research, talk at length with their oncologist, and make a decision that feels right for them.

After a few days of appointments, scans, meetings with the oncology surgery team and the plastic surgery team, it is time to head back to San Antonio. The huge plus is that the next day is Thanksgiving and David is home. He was originally supposed to be away for Thanksgiving. Silver linings. Our holiday is very quiet, low key, and lovely. It's just us and the girls. There is no

35

schedule…no rush.   It gives me enough quiet time to snap into focus all of the things for which I have to be grateful.

The next week is one of a thousand phone calls trying to get the earliest possible surgery date. This was more difficult than it sounds since it involved the coordination of the oncology team, the plastics team, and operating room availability. Throw in the holidays, and you've got a bit of a conundrum. In retrospect, the waiting was not that long. At the time, though, it felt an eternity. There was cancer growing inside of me, and I wanted it gone. The tumor felt like THE most unwelcome guest…like a houseguest who arrived in muddy boots, drank all of your beer, left crumbs in your carpet, said crass and inappropriate things in front of your kids, broke something expensive, farted and blamed the dog, and taught your toddler to twerk. Tumor: the kind of guest you want to bid farewell and never have return. I wanted it gone, gone, gone.

Finally, a surgery date…D-Day: December 11, 2012.

Three

Here We Go

December 2012

In the time between Thanksgiving and my mastectomy date, David returns to Afghanistan. I spent the time readying myself for surgery. I was able to buy some of the things I needed...a wedge pillow for the bed...loose button-down shirts...pillows for arm propping...essential oils to help ease things like nausea and anxiety...surgical bras....stretchy camisoles...and more. I wish I could say that preparing myself for surgery was as easy as simply shopping for some needed supplies.

It wasn't.

I needed to prime myself mentally and spiritually.

Faith can be such an important part of cancer treatment. My faith has seen me through many dark moments. If not for the hope that comes with faith, I would have been beyond lost during cancer. As for religions, I believe that unity of purpose of all world religions can advance mankind. If we could focus on the fundamental unity underlying all religions: oneness of humanity, elimination of prejudice, and harmony of science & religion....imagine how the world could be. No matter what sort of faith you practice, I believe we serve a just and benevolent God. A God we do not always understand, but one in which we have the faith that all things are for good. Something that really stood out to me at this point in my life was coined by author Phillip Yancey:

"I have learned to see beyond the physical reality in this world and to the spiritual reality. We tend to think, 'Life should be fair because God is fair.' But God is not life. And if I confuse God with the physical reality of life - by expecting constant good health, for example - then I set myself up for crushing disappointment. If we develop a relationship with God apart from our life circumstances, then we may be able to hang on when the physical reality breaks down. We learn to trust God, despite the unfairness of life."

I began to understand that circumstances did not have to be perfect in my life to feel joyful. No matter the challenges...

physical pain…financial woes…uncertain future…the fact is, we are all going to die. The questions are: How do I want to *live*? How do I *choose* to feel? I choose happiness. Cancer helped me discover that even in the midst of winter, there was inside of me an eternal summer if I chose to allow it.

That choice did not come without challenges, however. There would be times when choosing contentment took a little longer. And times when choosing contentment was downright hard. A particularly brutal trial was working through the difficultly of saying adios to my breasts. Since a mastectomy is often followed by reconstruction allowing a woman to appear "normal" in clothes, many people fail to realize that it is equivalent to an amputation. A part of your body is being cut from you. That part will never regenerate. Goodbye forever.

I have no doubt that a bilateral mastectomy was the right choice for me. I have never regretted it. It was; however, grueling to get through the thought that my breasts would be gone forever.

Sigh.

The gals. They made their debut between the summer of 8th and 9th grades….and they appeared almost overnight. I went from being teased for being absolutely flat chested to being teased for bursting out. (The teen years are awfully tough, right?!?!) The lady lumps and I became fast friends. We had a fun time filling out sweaters, prom dresses, and bikinis. New as they were, sometimes I was flummoxed by those frost detectors. How could boobs attract so much attention??? The sweater stretchers and I had a great time in college. So carefree. Fun we had; yes we did. *The* most *beautiful* thing we did together was nurse my girls.

Saying goodbye to them was going to be hard. I would never ever be able to feel sensation in the same way, if at all. They would never feel sensual beneath the brush of my lover's hands. They would never nurse another baby. They would never again be a soft place for my youngest (still my baby at age 2) to rest her head. They would never be quite the same.

But hey - its a free boob job, right? Wink wink.

I also spent the weeks leading up to my surgery getting physically ready. I am so thankful I discovered Pilates before my diagnosis. I have always been an exerciser, but to date, I had never fallen in love with any form of exercise the way I fell in love with Pilates. What is great about Pilates is that it can be modified for any and all fitness levels. A program can be designed to be challenging for anyone from beginning exercisers to professional athletes and everyone in between. It can also be extremely helpful in rehabilitating the body. As for women - or men- who go through breast surgery, specific Pilates exercises exist to help with healing and rehabilitation. Thankfully my Pilates mentor Jerilyn, a breast cancer survivor herself, was able to work with me before my surgery. The work helped me understand exactly what I would need to do post-operatively to target my specific needs. Exercise was paramount to my preparation and recovery throughout surgeries and chemotherapy. Movement has always helped me organize my ideas, motion taking care of emotion. It allowed me time to process my thoughts and quiet the frenzy of information running through me. So, I just kept moving and moving.

(My understanding of the need for *and* my love for stillness practiced through yoga would come later.)

Surgery time.

On Sunday December 9, my mom and dad arrive in San Antonio to take care of the girls. David arrives home from Afghanistan, and we take off to Houston. Monday is full of pre-op appointments. Blood draws for lab work. Meetings with my oncology surgery team. Meetings with my plastic surgery team.

Meetings with anesthesia. Even after all of this, it still seems surreal that in less than 24 hours, my breasts will be amputated. Luckily, I have a husband who keeps me laughing all day long. He gets my nerdy humor and isn't afraid to do corny things to crack me up. I love him.

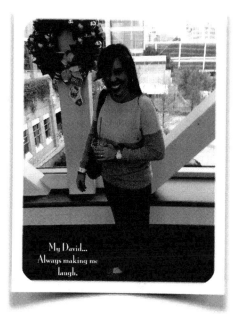

My David...
Always making me
laugh.

Surgery eve.

I have until midnight to keep eating, and I have been cleared for a glass of wine! Of course, David and I take full advantage and turn it into a date night. No kids….in a city with great eats….when in Rome! Dinner and drinks, here we come. Four a.m. is going to come early, but who cares…I will be in a coma most of the day anyway. Incredibly, Regina….one of my most dear friends in the whole wide world….is in town for business and is able to join us. We have a great time and share a lot of laughs over bidding my boobies bye-bye.

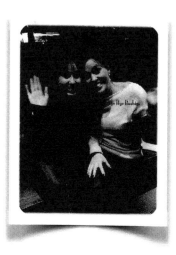

After dinner ends and we return to the hotel, the lightness of the mood shifts, and I find it nearly impossible to sleep. My emotions are torn between relief over removing the tumor from my body, anxiety over the surgery and recovery, and sadness over never feeling my breasts again. Thank God David is right by my side. His presence quells me. It always has, and I am certain it always will. He wraps me up in his strong arms and assures me that I will be the same me tomorrow that I am today.

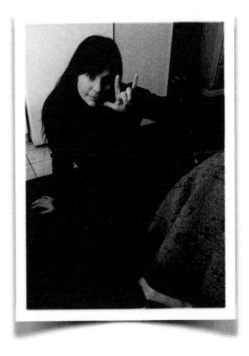

I am already awake when the alarm sounds signaling that it is time to hop up and shower. The getting dressed process is quick since there will be no makeup, jewelry, or cute ensemble to worry about. I ask David to take my wedding band with him so that he can place it on my finger as soon as I wake. I don't know why, but this is very important to me in that particular moment. I hate the naked feeling of my ring finger. Maybe it is that once I feel that wedding band back on my left hand, I will know that I've made it to the other side of surgery.

Our hotel is attached to the hospital, so we walk over and I check in for surgery. It is still dark outside. The halls are quiet, and the walk over is very surreal. We arrive at the admitting station, and it is abuzz with activity. I fill out some paperwork, then wait for my name to be called. The nurse who leads us to the admitting area is sweet as Tupelo honey. (Yay for no grumpy nurses!) He is also shorter than me, which probably puts him right around five feet tall. He also sounds IDENTICAL to Cleveland from Family Guy…. "OK Mrs. Holaaand. Right over there, you'll find your hospital gown, stockings, and socks. Once I go, you can remove everythaaang including your undergarments and slip those onnnnn," which conjures a thousand giggles from me and from David. (Yes, we both have the sense of humor of a 12 year old.)

I strip down and don the hospital couture....gown, cap, and support stockings...all sans undies... Sexxxxxxy! What a sight. Especially with my butt cheeks hanging out...which of course sends us into another fit of giggles as I streak around the room. I am sure some of the chortling is actually nervous laughter on my part, but laughs are welcome no matter what. People who don't find humor in life, especially during trying times, really baffle me. Gut-clenching laughter has to be one of my absolute favorite things ever! Laughter is a gift. When darkness begins to build inside, it is the light of laughter which casts it out. I find humor to be an essential element of a happy life. So get to giggling - and let go of taking life so seriously.

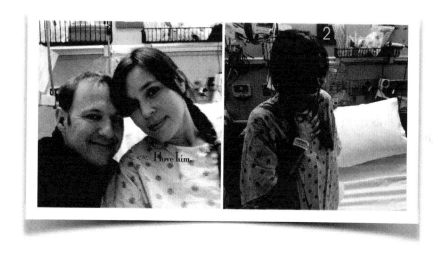

I settle into my bed. An IV is started. A million nurses, doctors, PAs, and anesthesiologists come by to each ask the same questions about my surgery. I guess it is to ensure they don't amputate a leg or something instead of my boobs. I do not mind though, as it is pretty important to feel confident that everyone is on the same page.

43

A priest stops by and asks if I would like him to pray with me. I answer with "Absolutely". His prayer is short and sweet, and it leaves me with the peace which passes all understanding. Appreciative.

Almost time now. Breathe in. Breathe out. Be strong. Be brave. They give me happy meds and I have just enough time to giggle some more before they wheel me down the hall. I kiss my David and off we go. I am barely hanging on when we reach the operating room. I am awake long enough to switch from the gurney to the operating table ....look around at the swirl of activity from the people and machines that surround me...and I am OUT.

Hours for which I am completely unaware pass, then I find myself struggling to wake. I have had few other operations before - and I loathe willing myself to wake and focus after anesthesia. My mind wakes first and the sensation of sound enters my ears. I want to open my eyes, but they are so heavy. It is like there is something dark and so, so, so heavy in my body pulling me just beneath the surface. I am not sure how much time passes in this purgatory, but I eventually open my eyes. My gaze finds my David, and I smile. At least I do in my mind. I have no idea if my facial muscles are cooperating or if I look dazed and confused. I probably look goofy as hell. I discover that I don't have to ask him for my wedding band; he has already placed it on my finger. Knowing that it is there soothes me.

My chest is bandaged. It will be several days before I am brave enough to look at what lies beneath. I am also equipped with four surgical drains: two on each side of my chest. Basically, each involves a tube sewn into my chest under my arms. Each tube is attached to a bulb that will collect fluid. The bulbs look like giant Christmas ornaments....so nice to know that I am en vogue for the holiday season! The bulbs will have to be drained twice a day until they are removed.

I have no idea how much time passes in recovery...it is a blur. My pain is apparent, but well managed, but I struggle with nausea and have to will myself not to vomit. I was given a scopolamine patch before surgery and pumped full of anti-nausea meds, but my nemesis found me still. The dose of meds is increased, and I am able to avoid puking...for now.

At some point, I am taken to a room. We settle in. Since my catheter has been removed, it isn't long until I reallllllly have to pee. I don't want to use the bedpan. I have lost so much modesty already, that I'd like to hang onto the small shred that remains. I am determined to make it to the restroom and wipe my own booty, but it does take David and a nurse to help me to there. It is maybe ten or fifteen steps form the bed to the toilet. It might as well be a thousand...because I nearly faint on the trip. I make it to the potty, and I am now almost certain that I am about to vomit. For some reason the nurse thinks that inhaling the scent of rubbing alcohol will help, so she shoves an alcohol pad under my nose and I GAG! (I am so regretting leaving my peppermint oil in the hotel room! It would have helped with the nausea, and it sure would have smelled better than rubbing alcohol.) OK. Breathe in. Breathe out. Focus. Do not puke. It will hurt so badly to puke. Don't do it! After a few minutes I compose myself and let them know that they can leave me seated and alone to tinkle. Thankfully, they agree and I summon them when I need help rising. I am beyond exhausted, but triumphant that I wiped my own arse! It is the little things.....

The night passes like any in a hospital. Short naps are interrupted by the whoosh of the compression contraptions....the checking of the vitals...the taking of the meds. Poor David is curled up on the chair-bed. He is attentive to my every need. I am a lucky girl.

Rise and shine. Time to nibble on something. Nausea is still plaguing me. I am able to eat a bit thanks to Phenergan. It has been less than 24 hours since my boobs were lopped off, and now it is time to get up and walk. Game face: ON. A waltz down the hall and around the nurses' station will be attempted. My friend Jeanne's dad had spent time at MDA, and he referred to the trek as the MD Anderson Marathon. So apt! I have no idea how long it took me, but I made it…one little shuffling step at a time.

My doctors come by for a visit and to discharge me. We head back to the hotel where we will be staying for a few more days until I am able to tolerate the three hour drive home. The wheelchair ride from the hospital to the entrance of the hotel ranges from comical to down right scary…the guy wheeling me is a speed demon. I am relieved when David initiates a takeover!

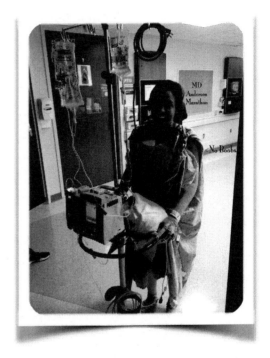

The remainder of the day is spent in and out of sleep. Apparently, some of the day is spent purchasing and reading magazines on my iPad. I remember none of this…I discovered the purchases at a later date…and reread the magazines. Glad I didn't venture to shop online! Note: drugs and shopping do not mix.

The next morning my old foe, nausea, is back in full force. This time…it wins. Yikes. I cannot quite describe the pain that accompanies vomiting with a chest full of sutures and surgical drains. It is probably the most physically painful thing I have ever experienced. The hotel is equipped with a shower stool which David positions in front of the toilet for me. Then I ask him to leave the room - I don't want him seeing his bride this way. Though he would gladly hold my hand and my hair for the whole event, I just don't want him to see my face contorting or my body writhing. I don't want to cause him more pain by watching my tears fall because I feel absolutely defeated. In this moment, cancer is making mincemeat of me.

In sickness and in health. That man meant what he vowed.

Calls are made to the doctor, and David makes another trip to the pharmacy. Thankfully, by the end of the day, we find the best combo of nausea meds to stop the vomiting. I am even able to nibble a bit and keep it down. Sweet relief.

Another day or so (I honestly cannot remember if it was one, two, or three more days since I was in a drug-induced haze), and I am fit to make the ride home. (Speaking of drug-induced hazes, I could never make it as an addict....I hate, hate, hate, feeling that disconnected from life.) David helps me downstairs and to the car. He insulates me with pillows and buckles me up for the ride home. I am elated at the thought of seeing our girls.

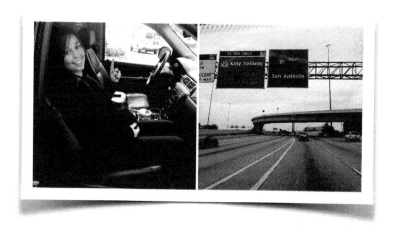

I feel every single bump along I-10 from Houston to San Antonio. Each. And. Every. One. Big. Or. Small. (My recurring thought is: Oh dear Lord....we have to make this same trip back in a few days for my first post op visit.) Finally, we arrive home.

47

The girls race to the car to meet us. I did not do the best job of preparing them for the sight of my surgical drains, perhaps because I had no idea how cumbersome they would be or what they would actually look like. Sarah Jayne opens my door and leans in to hug me....gently. She sees the drains, and then she quickly averts her eyes in an attempt to hide her look of anguish. That kills me.

The first thing Genevieve (2 at the time) wants me to do is hold her, but it will be weeks before I am able. Again, I die a little on the inside.

Damn cancer and all that it tries to steal.

We spend a few days at home. They pass in a blur. My post-op exercise program consists of shuffling from one room to the next and doing a few very MINOR post-op Pilates stretches. Oh- and at this point I would consider showering and getting dressed (with help from David since I couldn't do it by myself yet) part of my exercise program as well because it was dang hard!

Speaking of showering and being naked...it was during this time that I finally made myself look in the mirror sans bandages. I guess I would say that the experience was breathtaking. Not so much in a breathtakingly beautiful way, but more of a gasping for air to steady my emotions kind of way.

My breasts were...gone.

In their place, there was bruised, swollen, disfigured, and stitched skin. Tubes were sewn into my sides draining blood and lymph into bulbs. It was grotesque. I allow myself to cry and grieve for a bit. Then: Breathe in. Breathe out. Be brave. Heal.

I have shared that nausea was my biggest foe, and I would have to say that surgical drains came in a close second. They (all four of them) had to be stripped, drained, and cleaned twice a day. Stripping involved holding the tube where they were sewn into my body between two fingers with one hand and using the other hand to pinch and slide an alcohol soaked square down the length of the tube. (If alcohol entered the incision site....it would make me wince and gasp for air because of the pain. Yikes.) Then the bulb was opened and drained into a measuring cup and the volume was recorded. The amount of daily volume would determine when the drains could be removed. David would perform this twice daily duty for me. Bless him.

Here comes some comic relief. (About time, right?!?!) I was standing topless in the bathroom as David tended my drains. Genevieve wanders in and looks at my chest....and she looks really puzzled. Then she cocks her head to the side and says, "Mommy, your boobies look funny". I laughed and questioned, "They do?". She replies, "Yes, they look like they popped. Popped balloons.". I died laughing, because they did in fact look just like popped, wrinkly, strangely colored balloons! Out of the mouths of babes....leave it to toddlers to keep it real.

David and I return to MDA for my first post op visits with my surgeons. I arrive looking pretty normal in my baggy shirt. Underneath I am full of stitches and a tool apron is holding my drains. Party on the outside, Schneider from One Day At A Time underneath.

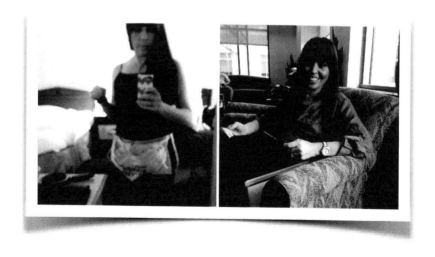

As for my chest, what still looks like Frankenstein to me apparently looks "great" to my doctors. That is good news. More good news: two of my drains can be removed. Yippppeeeeee! The process is pretty quick, but not painless. It involves clipping the stitches around the tubing...then with a deep breath...pulling out the tube. (I'd say the portion that was inside of me was about a foot long.) The pain is sharp and intense but over quickly. So now I am down to two drains and the remaining two "Christmas Ornament" drain bulbs are replaced with smaller "hand grenade" bulbs. My plastic surgeon gives David the clear to remove my remaining drains when the drainage volume reaches the right level. This is great news since we plan to travel to Alabama for Christmas. David did spend many, many years as a Special Forces Combat Medic...Drains: no biggie for an 18D! I trust him completely and inherently.

Next stop: oncology surgeon. He will deliver the pathology results and the results of the sentinel node biopsy. Based on the biopsy that revealed aggressiveness of my tumor, my oncologist has already recommended chemotherapy. (Some people do not know whether they will need chemo until they know whether or not they are node positive.) Still, we are hoping for negative lymph nodes simply because that would indicate a better prognosis. First, the surgeon and his team take a look at my chest. They too think it looks grrrreatttttt. Cool. FYI - I have zero modesty any more. I have lost count of how many times my chest has been looked at, poked, smooshed, touched, imaged, photographed, etc. They really should give out Mardi Gras beads to breast cancer patients.

Now for the surgical pathology report and the node results. The pathology report confirms that I am ER/PR + and HER2-. It also reveals that I have invasive mammary carcinoma with mixed ductal and lobular features. This means I have both IDC and ILC. Unfortunately, the report also reveals that cancerous cells were found in my lymph nodes. Dayyyyyyum. Damn, damn, damn.

However, the amount of cancer in my nodes is not overwhelming. Of ten nodes removed, only three are positive.

This news sets the stage for more decision making. Do I keep my remaining nodes or have all of them in the area removed? I am already at risk for lymphedema (forever and ever and ever). My risk for it and the severity of it will rise if I have all of them removed. However, the only way to know if the remaining nodes are clear is to have them removed and tested. Decisions, decisions.

I'd rather be making last-minute Christmas shopping decisions.

Both my oncology surgeon and my oncologist explain (using a mathematically derived prediction) that there is around a 90% chance that the remaining nodes will be clear. On the surface, that seems like a great number....but for the girl who had a 0.3% chance of developing breast cancer in her thirties and snagged it anyway....that number is not as reassuring as it should be. Since chemo targets cancer cells, the idea is that IF there are errant cancer cells, chemo should eradicate them. I decide against another surgery to remove all of the nodes. That area of my body has already been greatly compromised, and I'd like to keep the few remaining axillary nodes.

All in all, though not perfect, a very good day.

We make the three hour trip back to San Antonio, and pack our bags since we are flying to Alabama the next day. At this point, you may be thinking I am nuts to fly 1000 miles away ten days after a bilateral mastectomy. The thing is, I was mentally bent on making the trip. Cancer takes so much from you. Little things like showering, laughing with your kids, taking a walk around the block, and keeping plans....all the little 'normal' things of life.....feel like great victories. So crazy or not, keeping those plans made me feel a little victorious.

My mom is still in San Antonio with us. She stays with me while David and Sarah Jayne slip away to run some errands. When they return, David presents me with a small box....small enough and of the shape to suggest only one thing: jewelry! I open it, and he has taken my engagement ring and had it reset in a very beautiful way. He says he wants me to know that he would marry me all over again. I swoon.

Flying with drains.

I have no idea what to expect, and I am hoping that it won't be a big deal. I decide my best bet will be to just confess to TSA as we head through security. It turns out to be just fine. The TSA lady lets me know that after I pass through the scanners, I will have to touch my drains and have my fingers swabbed for explosives. No biggie. Everything was hidden beneath a nice, cute, flowing cardigan. Before walking through the metal detector, though, I am instructed to remove said camouflaging cardigan. DANG!!! There I stand....in my camisole....completely flat chested with drains bulging. In my mind, I may as well have shown up totally NEKKID, because that is how exposed I feel. It is all in my head, though, as all the people surrounding me are lost in their own shuffle trying to make sure they leave security with their shoes...jewelry... bags...ID... computer....children.... At least if anyone was shocked by my appearance, no one pointed and laughed.

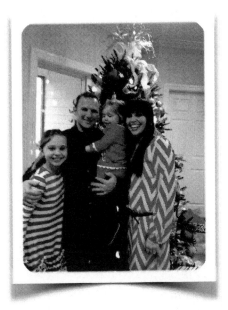

We spend the holidays with family and friends. I am

able to soak in my mom and dad and my sisters and nephews. David is able to remove my remaining drains on Christmas Eve... MERRY CHRISTMAS TO ME! Christmas Day is perfect. I am surrounded by family, and the day is filled with love and laughter.

David has to fly out the next day to return to Afghanistan. BoooooooooHooooooooo. He will return for the start of chemotherapy at the beginning of February. I am grateful that he was unexpectedly home for the holidays even if it did take cancer to make that happen.

I am also thankful that cancer - like any of life's immense challenges - is helping me appreciate that the important things in life are love, family, friendships, bonds, and peace of mind....the kind of peace of mind not based on circumstances, because circumstances certainly change.

Four

Transition

January is spent recovering from surgery, beginning the expansion process, and preparing for chemo. Exercise helped with all of this. During this time, exercise was not at all about being thinner or striving for a perfect body. It was about recovering, building strength, and clearing & sharpening my mind. It was about dedication even when I felt down and out. It was about dragging myself to the gym even when I felt uncomfortable with my physical disfigurement. It was about pushing through the physical and emotional pain to gain a deeper strength…one far deeper than I knew existed. It was about regaining what cancer was trying to steal from me. TAKE THAT, CANCER….POW!

My exercise program consisted of walking and Pilates. Why Pilates? So many reasons! I first became interested in Pilates because of back and hip pain from some old injuries. I knew that Pilates focused on core strength and spinal alignment, and that by achieving those, many maladies could be remedied. The deeper I dug, though, I realized it was much more. The Pilates Method, when practiced correctly, is a powerful mind-body program incorporating quality breathing to achieve a strong, well-balanced, flexible body without creating bulk. It can create a long and lean body with slender and toned thighs and abdomen. Welllll…..who wouldn't want that? Yes, please!! Pilates isn't meditative in the same way that Yoga is. I find it meditative and soothing in its own way, though. Focusing

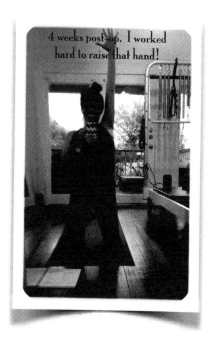

4 weeks post-op. I worked hard to raise that hand!

on isolating the right muscles at the right time to achieve the movements leaves little room for other thoughts to buzz around in your head....which equals serenity for me.

Motion takes care of emotion.

The method was begun by Joseph Pilates. He has a fascinating life story. Long story short: he was born in Germany... immigrated to England in 1912 where he taught self defense to detectives of the Scotland Yard...was placed in internment camp at the outbreak of WWI during which time he created exercise rehabilitation programs for wounded warriors by rigging springs to hospital beds...War ends and he returns to Germany where officials ask him to teach his fitness method to the German army....which prompts him to leave for good. He immigrated to the US in 1926....opened a studio in NYC with his wife Clara... ran the studio until his death in 1967. His work is carried on by several of the students whom he mentored through the years. These students went on to open their own studios. My favorite of these students is Eve Gentry.

When Eve was diagnosed with breast cancer and had a radical mastectomy in 1955, she was devastated that she could no longer lift her arms. (A radical mastectomy not only involves removal of the breast tissue, but also all of the axillary lymph nodes along with the pectoralis major and pectoralis minor muscles.) Anyone would be crushed, but Eve was a professional dancer. She couldn't imagine no longer dancing. In hopes that he could help, she solicited assistance from Joe. Want to know what his response to her plea for help was? "Don't worry. We fix." And fix they did! She made a full recovery and was able to perform advanced exercises with power and grace. Footage of their achievement was submitted for review by doctors at a local hospital. Joe was seeking endorsement of his program so that it could be used to help others. The doctors accused Joe of lying as it was "impossible" to make such a recovery after a radical mastectomy. Not one to give up, Joe persisted. Want to know what came next? I LOVE THIS PART…..they re-shot the footage. Only this time, Eve was topless. Yasssssssssss, girl! Oh how I love a good comeback story. Sadly, the doctors still rejected his method of recovery therapy as Joe did not have a medical degree. (Sound familiar of alternative and complementary therapies even today?) Eve returned to professional dancing and later established the Gentry technique. She died in 1994 at the age of 84 years.

Okay, okay….I could talk Pilates forever! I urge you to try it. If it isn't your forte, though, know this: your body's ability to heal is greater than anyone has ever led you to believe. Find some sort of physical activity that you love, and get moving. Channel your inner strength and show everyone who is boss!

So….January. Exercise and prepping for chemo. The fear of the unknown was a beast of burden. How sick would I feel? Would the actual infusion hurt? Could I take care of my family? Would I *really* lose my hair? When? What other side effects would I experience?

What else was happening in January? Friendships were shifting. I had read that after a cancer diagnosis, some friends would bail on you. This sounded absolutely absurd to me. Ludicrous. How could a friend desert someone in their time of great need? Well, they weren't lying….it happens! I had a few "fringe friends" who just sort of faded away…but I had one dear friend who just disappeared. POOF! Gone. Baffling. In the same breath, I was blessed with tons of wonderful friends…old and new. So many people who watched out for me, from near and far. My sisters, Jennifer and Sally, who sent cheer through the mail. So many kind souls who said the nicest things and offered prayers and positive vibes for me. So many who happily did favors for me. Brought coffee. Gifted me things. (My thank you list here is extensive.) Watched my kids (THANK YOU mom & dad, Louisa, Heather, Whitney, Ashley, and Kate). Picked up meds. Let me cry. Laughed with me. Listened while I talked.

If someone you love is diagnosed with cancer, please don't disappear. Be a good friend. If you don't know what being a good friend means, it is simple really. *Just be there.* Don't worry about having all the "right things" to say. Sometimes there really are no words. Your presence can be enough. Holding space is enough. Friends multiply the good things in life and divide the evils. I will forever be grateful for the people who showed me so many kindnesses. It is my prayer that I will somehow be able to pay all of it forward.

Sidebar: Upon editing this chapter, I did think of some doozies that were said to me. Know that sometimes it is hard to find the "right words" - and that is ok! Just do your best. However, these are some of the things that you can just go ahead and NOT SAY ever to someone diagnosed with cancer:

- "At least you got the good cancer." (Wait, what? There is some *good* cancer that I don't know about?)
- "I'd just tell my doctor to just lop 'em off and be done with it." (Mmmmhhhhmmmm....as if it is just that easy. Also, lopping them off doesn't assure that the cancer won't return.)
- "At least you get a new pair!" (Yes, indeed. After many grueling surgeries. And they will be prosthetic. They won't feel a thing.)
- "I know exactly how you feel." (Probably not...unless you, too, have/had cancer.)
- "Cancer is a gift." (Of course good things can come from cancer, but I don't think there is anyone out there asking Santa for a cancer diagnosis.)
- "At least you'll get some down time with surgeries and chemo." (Ummm....no words. Other than, are you kidding me?!)

I am sure that I could think of a few more, but you get the gist. Take note and carry on.

At this point in my treatment plan, once I am dressed and made up, I look pretty normal. Clothes hide much. Anyone who didn't know me would not have guessed what was beneath my baggy tunics...or how much it hurt...or how exhausting daily chores were. This scenario often left me annoyed by others. Prime example: at the grocery store I am given the stink eye several times for not moving my cart fast enough and for taking forever to load my groceries and kids into the car. Here I am...feeling so accomplished for simply doing my own shopping...with kids....three weeks post mastectomy....and here was some fool trying to ruin it by waiting for my parking space...blinker flashing...fingers impatiently tap, tap, tapping on the steering wheel...as I try to get my things into the car. For a moment I consider flashing her, but I fear the old bag may faint. So, I breathe in...breathe out....and shake off the negativity she is bringing...finish loading my car at my own snail's pace....and head on my way....head held high.

The remainder of January is spent traveling back and forth to MDA for the expansion process. Recall that during my mastectomy surgery, expanders were placed behind my pectoralis muscles in my chest. To make room for permanent implants, these muscles would have to be stretched over time. So, once a week for the month of January, here is how it went. David was still in Afghanistan...Maggie would be at her mom's house...I would arrange for Sarah Jayne to sleep over at a friend's house (McGinlay family....couldn't have done it without you! Genevieve and I would load up and make the three hour trek to Houston. We would stay overnight in a hotel...during which time my toddler became very accustomed to room service...ha! It was such a treat for her and so funny to see her pick up the menu and pretend to read it, say "Service, please", and tell me what she wanted. (Again, it's the little things, right?) The next day, I'd go to my appointment and Genevieve would stay at the childcare center provided by MDA. (How incredible is it that MDA has a daycare for the children of patients?)

Appointment time. Just *how* do they do the expansion….you may be wondering. It is crazy and fascinating. At least it is to me. The expanders are saline filled bags equipped with metal ports. The port is palpable, but to ensure correct placement for the needle, a little device that is just like a stud finder is used. The stud finder is placed on your chest and it pinpoints the port. Next, a big ass needle which is attached to tubing and a large vial of saline is inserted through the skin and muscle into the port. The plunger is pushed and saline solution enters the expanders. It may be 50ccs, 100ccs, or whatever variation the doctor or physician's assistant deems appropriate at the time. It is beyond bizarre to look down and literally see your chest grow!

My first expansion wasn't painful at all. I felt a little pressure and tightness along with a tugging sensation, but that was about it. My subsequent fills were not so pain-free, however. I'd say my remaining fills were godawful. The pain would hit on my drive home to San Antonio. I swear I thought that my pecs were being torn from my breastbone and that my rhomboids were being ripped from my spine. Holy hell it hurt! I learned that muscle relaxers helped tremendously. Some women have shared that expansions were only mildly uncomfortable for them…others that it was miserably painful. I suppose it depends on your anatomy and how many ccs they pump into you at a time. Fun times.

I went for weekly expansion sessions so that most of my fills would be achieved before chemo started.

Sometime during this time frame, I cut my locks from super long to pixie short. I figured a preemptive short cut would prepare me for the baldness that was to come. I'd never really worn my hair short. Okay…I did once…in 7th grade…before I had boobs…and I was mistaken for a boy. TWICE! So, I shied away from short dos from that point forward. But here I found myself again…boob-less with short hair. Anyone else hear the universe laughing?! Bahahahahaha….I had to laugh too!

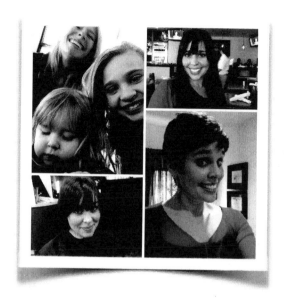

The month of January was full of ups and downs. Mentally, I faced many fears. When those fears became a bit overwhelming, I'd allow myself a good cry. Sometimes I wanted nothing more than to stick my head in the sand and pretend there was no cancer. Alas, there was no crawling under the covers and making it all go away forever. No pretending it never happened. Only small steps forward. Unexpected laughs. New found strengths. Mirrors that did not matter.

Like any major trial, cancer changes you. You enter the battle as one person, then you are forged by challenge after challenge into a new version of yourself. If you allow it, you are molded into something stronger. Wiser. Braver. More thankful. Better.

Five

Chem-Oh-No

February, March, April 2013

Perhaps you have noticed that to this point, each chapter has been dedicated to a single month. The chemo months are lumped together because that is exactly how the time passed -in one, big, lumped-together, blurry haze.

CHEMO 1

David arrives home again. His presence instantly makes me feel lighter and brings extra joy for me and for the girls. We have all done the "daddy is home; daddy is deployed" thing so many times that the transition is quick.

Chemo number one has arrived, and it is time to head to the START Cancer center. We stop on the way to grab a coffee from our favorite coffee shop: Local Coffee. I opt for an iced latte. (I do this again for every chemo infusion.....and to this day....I cannot handle an iced latte. I think I ruined them forever! But, I still adore the coffee from Local Coffee. In fact, 90% of this book was penned there.)

I am babbling now....maybe trying to avoid the topic of chemo....still gives me the willies! OK. Back to chemo....I head to the appointment equipped with my Big Bag of Fun: a cozy blanket to keep me warm...peppermint oil for my nausea...water for hydration and flushing out chemo toxins...iPad....magazines...kindle....snacks. I feel prepared, and feeling prepared helps me feel calm. (Truth be told about the Bag of Fun...I wound up using the water and the blanket, but David kept me laughing and entertained the whole time, so I didn't really need all that stuff. Ashley Williams and Ashley Farless, if y'all are reading, my packed bag would have made you proud! This girl was over packed and extra prepared.)

We arrive and sign in. Soon I am called to the treatment room. It is sun-drenched. There is a flurry of activity. I am the youngest person there. It feels odd to look around and realize I am in the mix with some who look as if they are knocking on death's door. I don't say that with any disrespect. It is really just a keen observation. I wonder if some of them will make it to their next infusion date. Not everyone looks that way, but I cannot help but notice those who do. It is unsettling, and it makes me sad.

First order of business (and every girl's favorite): weigh in. Next up: choose your chair for the day. Then temperature and blood pressure are taken. (BP in the left arm now and forever....no BP or vein sticks in the right since nodes were removed.) One of my favorite things (NOT!) happens next: an IV is started. (Many people undergoing chemo have a port for access placed in their chest. My oncologist thought that my veins looked so nice that I wouldn't need one. Mmmmhhhhmmmm...I have learned that judging veins by the way they look is right up there with judging a book by its cover.) Now, I don't mind shots so much, but I LOATHE IVs. I hate the feeling that accompanies digging for a vein. My veins are tricky. Surrrrre, they look easy to stab, but they tend to roll. Always. Several attempts later, a successful IV line is established. First, blood is drawn and sent for a quick check to ensure that my blood counts are good enough to receive chemo that day. A little time passes and counts are deemed good.

Showtime.
Here. We. Go.

Breathe in. Breathe out. This is the stuff that should clean house. It'll wipe out any remaining, stealth, mean cancer cells. Breathe in. Breathe out. I. Can. Do. This.

Even before the first chemo drip, my senses are sent reeling. The IV line is flushed, and for me, there is an immediate and peculiar taste in my mouth. It tastes like rubbing alcohol....as if I am temporarily drowning in it as the sensation fills my nose and mouth. It is nasty and overwhelming, but thankfully, pretty short-lived. It is my first experience with senses that will remain in overdrive throughout the chemo months with some effects

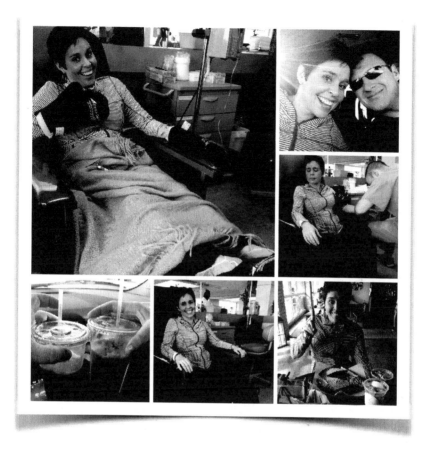

lingering far longer. Smells, light, and sound will all seem amplified. I am first pumped full of pre-meds. Antihistamines. Anti-nausea meds. Steroids. Then a bag of saline is run to flush the line. My first chemo drug is hooked up next: Taxotere. It is notorious for causing problems in the hands and feet: burned skin, black nails which eventually fall off, and permanent neuropathy. My doctor has found success with icing the hands and feet during infusion to prevent such afflictions. So, for the hour that Taxotere drips and travels through my veins, my hands and feet are placed in frozen "gloves" and "socks". Talk about an intense feeling. Geeeeeeeeeezzzzzzzz! I power through it, though. I'd like to avoid permanent nerve damage if possible. An hour later, the Taxotere drip is complete. I lose the ice packs and receive another bag of saline to flush the line. Next in the lineup: Cytoxan. It drips for an hour, followed by another bag of saline. The whole ordeal has lasted nearly five hours, and we are done for the day.

David and I leave and celebrate with a late lunch. The idea was a great one...at first. Later, I regret it as I toss my cookies. I learned to munch more on bland things *during* the infusions which seemed to help the nausea somewhat.

For the next few days, I am tired, achy, and a bit nauseated. My tastebuds change. Most things taste like burned toast. Mouthwash tastes like melted crayons. A red, raised, itchy rash appears.

Meanwhile, life rocks on. Maggie and Sarah Jayne are busy with school. Genevieve is busy being a toddler. I try to walk, do Pilates, and rest as much as I can.

We return to the doctor one week later for labs and a checkup. Chemo targets rapidly dividing cells. Since it cannot differentiate between rapidly dividing cancer cells and rapidly dividing healthy cells, it wreaks havoc on many things including white blood cells, red blood cells, etc. A CBC (complete blood count) is performed to see how my body is faring, and to determine if it is faring well enough to avoid a shot called Neulasta (pegfilgrastin). This shot is used to treat neutropenia (a lack of the specific white blood cells called neutrophils) in cancer patients. It stimulates the bone marrow to produce WBCs. Sometimes, Neulasta is automatically prescribed for the day following chemo infusion. However, because it can have some pretty uncomfortable side effects, and because some insurance companies will not cover it unless it has been proven (by a round of chemo that knocks your CBC levels too low) to be needed, often doctors will wait until after the first round of chemo to determine if you need it.

Back to the doctor visit. We chat a minute about my rash and about how I am feeling. He prescribes something for the rash. Then we talk blood work. I want to know if my counts earned me an "A+. Admittedly, I am a girl who loves an "A"! With a hearty laugh, he tells me that I did not make the Dean's List. In fact, I earned a lot of "F" scores. My counts were wiped out.

Per the Mayo Clinic, normal ranges look something like this for a normal, adult female:
RBC: 3.9-5.03 trill cells/L
HgB: 12.0-15.5 g/dL
Hct: 34.9-44.5%
WBC: 3.5-10.5 bill cells/L
ANC 1.7-4

My RBC, HgB, and Hct levels were 3.5, 10, and 30 respectively. Low, but not terribly bad. My WBC level was 1 and my ANC (absolute neutrophil count) was 0.17. POINT ONE SEVEN. Yikes. This put me at great risk for infection for not being able to fight off anything I may contract. So, the doctor places me on antibiotics and an anti-fungal and gives me meds for my rash. Then he sends me on my way until my next chemo in two weeks.

Another week passes, and my scalp begins to itch like crazy. Uh-oh. Here it comes. I had been dreading this part, and I had secretly hoped that I'd experience a chemo anomaly and somehow keep my locks. My hair had long been my security blanket....my cape. A passage from Hemingway's "A Farewell to Arms" kept popping in my head as I thought of losing my hair:

"I loved to take her hair down and she sat on the bed and kept very still, except suddenly she would dip down to kiss me while I was doing it, and I would take out the pins and lay them on the sheet and it would be loose and I would watch her while she kept very still and then take out the last two pins and it would all come down and she would drop her head and we would both be inside of it, and it was the feeling of inside a tent or behind a falls. She had wonderfully beautiful hair and I would lie sometimes and watch her twisting it up in the light that came in the open door and it shone even in the night as water shine sometimes just before it is really daylight."

Sigh.

Losing my hair would also signal to the world: sick person! Cancer patient! I did not really feel ready for that, but the tingling of my scalp screamed, "Get ready....its time!". Over the next day or so, the tingling gave way to clumps of hair on my pillow...hair in the shower...hair leaving a trail behind me. Hair everywhere. Breathe in. Breathe out. Take control.

Cancer had taken my breasts, and now it was taking my hair. But— I had a choice in *how* it would take my hair. At any given moment in life, we have the power to say: Wait! This is not how my story is going to go. I can switch it up. I have a choice in this matter. As for my hair, it was going, but I wasn't going to let it go strand by agonizing strand.

Out with the clippers. Sarah Jayne had said for weeks that when it was time, she wanted to shave my head. I was totally for it! So, we plugged in the clippers, and I took my seat. She was excited at first, but when it came time to put those clippers to my head, she said, "Mama, I just can't do it.". She was scared. Secretly, I was a little reluctant, too...but I wanted to follow

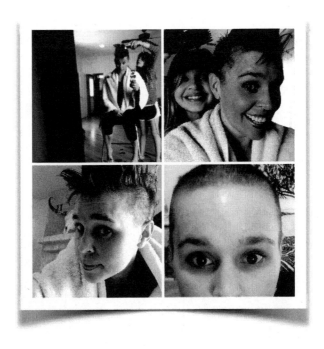

through and take control. I told Sarah Jayne that it was okay, then I took the clippers and made the first pass. Buzzzzzzzzzz. Once the ice was broken, she jumped in and gave me a mohawk. We laughed a lot. Once I was bald, I did feel liberated….my hair was gone on my terms. Sweet Genevieve then asked when would it be her turn for a shave. A bald head means nothing in the eyes of a two year old. Why then should it matter to me? (Not gonna lie, though….it would be weeks and weeks before I was brave enough to go commando in public.)

David was out of town for work when we had the shaving party. As with many events in our family, he was able to join in via FaceTime. (Where would we be without technology?) He arrived home a few days later and told me that he found me beautiful as a baldie. The next afternoon, the house grew suspiciously quiet… and with a houseful of kids, you always know something is brewing when it is quiet. Then I heard giggles coming from one of the bathrooms. There, I find David with all three girls. He had let them shave his head completely bald. We were now twins!

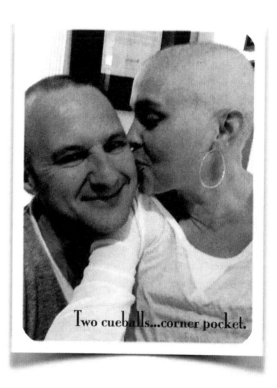
Two cueballs...corner pocket.

David is my best friend and my confidant. This man with whom I laugh…share my secrets…confide my hopes, dreams, fears, and frustrations…who lends a patient ear and sage advice. This man who, in our moments filled with joy, helps me find a place where I am completely free. Though I am disfigured and bald, this man still kisses me out of desire, not consolation. I am a fortunate girl indeed.

Let's talk for a few about being bald. The whole experience served as a good reminder that control is an illusion. I always suspected that the hair on our heads was put there to remind us of that very thing. From straighteners to pomades to curlers to colors…try as we may…it is often hard to control what kind of hair day we are having. Losing it all revealed a realization that sometimes you just have to let go of the reins.

That wasn't the only lesson I learned from being bald. Here is a funny one….several years before, I had gotten a very small tattoo on my neck at the base of my hairline. (Sarah Jayne's initials formed into a little heart.) I chose that spot because I knew that I could show it when I wished since I would ALWAYS have hair to cover it for work situations and whatnot. Well. Ultimatums like "Always" fall in the same category with things like "Never". If a thought with one of those words so much as runs through my head, I am going to be proven wrong. It is like a Murphy's Law of sorts…..Natalie's law. I have learned not to make statements aloud containing "Never" or "Always"….and I am starting to think I should banish any *thoughts* that contain either word, too, since such thoughts may have the same effect as thinking of the Stay Puft Marshmallow Man in Ghostbusters. If you think it…it will happen.

The next baldie lesson I learned was that you can, in fact, simultaneously be both the most interesting (as evidenced by stares) and the most invisible (verified by lightening fast averted gazes) person in the room. I have spent most of my life as a generally liked, warm, and plugged-in person. Being bald helped me understand what it feels like to be an outsider. So many times I could feel eyes boring holes through me. When I would look to meet someone's gaze with a smile, their head would snap in the other direction so quickly that I am shocked no one experienced whiplash. More than once, I overheard people say things like, "Do you think that is a fashion statement?" or "Do you think she has… whisper…gasp…cancer?".

Let me offer some advice here. If you are ever busted staring at a baldie…or someone who is physically different…or whatever….don't turn away. Simply offer a "Hi" or "Hello" or "How are you today?". Or—You don't have to say anything at all; you can just give a smile. You have no idea how far your kindness may go. One night during my bald days, I was standing in line at the Purple Garlic to pick up dinner. There I was in my scarf. My head may have been hanging a little low as I was learning it was easier to just avoid eye contact than endure looks of pity and averting eyes…which has a way of eventually making you feel sort of invisible. The lady behind me struck up a conversation by telling me that she loved my pretty scarf. I thanked her and laughingly told her that it was hiding a very bald head. She said she had figured as much but she thought I looked beautiful all the same. We laughed more and chatted until I picked up my order. As I headed to my car, I was moved to tears. I had felt so ignored in public as of late - so insignificant and invisible - that those few kinds words struck a chord in me and turned me into an emotional, blubbering mess.

The worst offenders of the stare-then-ignore crowd were women around my age at my gym. The older people were far more kind and more likely to speak to me. The thirty-something and forty-something set…they were downright awful! Did they find me akin to Medusa, thinking that if they looked at me and I looked back that they would catch cancer? It bothered me for a while, but then it became a bit of a comical challenge to see if anyone would speak to me. Not many did, so I just proudly donned my "yes they're fake…my real ones tried to kill me" tank, did my workout, and had my own laughs. I wasn't about to let stares make me feel uncomfortable enough to keep me at home. I am so glad I didn't, because it was a trip to the gym that led me to an amazing friend exactly when I needed it. I would swear our friendship was a divine match. Molly…thirty something bad ass super mom. Same college degree as me: check! Appreciates exercise: check! Army wife: check! Has a toddler: check! Zest for life: check! Cancer (brain): check! Our conversations flow easily from potty training to cancer treatments to travel and more.

Serendipity at its finest.

CHEMO 2

A few days pass, and it is time for round two. Chemo day is filled with much of the same…trouble finding a vein, steroids, saline drips, chemo drips, iced hands and feet. On the up side, David is there to entertain me and make me laugh. It is like a day date.

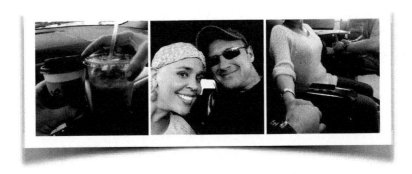

The next day, I receive a Neulasta shot to stimulate my bone marrow in hopes of maintaining decent blood counts. Over the next several days, I learn that when it comes to a chemo-hangover, there is no cure from the hair of the dog that bit you! The effects of round two are more intense than round one and they last longer. This will be the trend as chemo progresses.

Now, no one is going to mistake chemotherapy drugs for party drugs though I am sure they kill just as many brain cells. I had read about "chemo brain" (a real, scientific thing), but I didn't think much about it until it hit me. OhhhhEmmmmGeeee. Talk about a fuzzy brain…I became so forgetful! (The worst offense was probably leaving my new iPad on top of the car and driving away…where it promptly slid off…crashed into the road…and slipped into a storm drain. Oopsie! Did I mention I have THE most understanding husband in the world?!?!) I had a HORRIBLE time recalling words. Simple things like "toaster" or "acrobat"… I'd be in the middle of a conversation, and I would have to stop mid-sentence because I couldn't find the word I wanted to say. It was endlessly frustrating to me. That chemo brain still makes an appearance from time to time, though it has improved greatly.

A week passes…in a blur…and it is time for David to return to Afghanistan. Again. A bit of anxiety creeps in, as it always does each time he deploys. I wonder how I will do it all without him. What will I do without his help…his humor… his support? What will I do without this amazing man who looked at me today and emphatically declared "You're beautiful!". (I know that at this point, I clearly look like Uncle Fester: bald..swollen face..dark under-eye circles. The only thing missing is a lightbulb in my mouth…and he is still telling me that I am pretty.) "I will miss everything about you while I am away. I will miss the way you smell. I will miss the way your

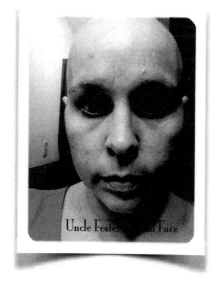

Uncle Fester's Face

body folds so perfectly into mine. I will miss kissing your eyelids. I will miss your smile lighting the room."

Sighhhhhhh.
I miss him already.

Off he goes and oh-blah-dee oh-blah-dah, life goes on...
Make no mistake. Life does not slow down for cancer.
Pre-teen drama to sort. Baby booties to wipe. Meals to prepare.
Laundry to wash. Groceries to buy. Toilets to plunge. Messes to
clean. Homework. Doggie to feed. Carpools to drive. You
know....life. Some days it feels like I am riding my bicycle uphill.
A tall, sandy hill. And the chain just fell off.

Good thing Ashley Farless is coming all the way from
Chattanooga soon.

Ashley Farless....sista from another mista. College friend,
sorority sister, and roommate. Mama Farless...that is what we
called her in college because you could always count on her to take
care of you. Friend through thick and thin. Godmother to my
children. Love her more than my shoe collection. She is going to
make round 3 so much better.

CHEMO 3

Treatment day goes like the others...trouble with the
vein...steroids...saline...chemo...blah, blah, blah. My weigh-in
shows that I have gained weight. You read that right: *gained
weight.* Awesome. So lovely that you can basically eat nothing
but air for three weeks and GAIN weight from steroids. Thanks
cancer, your gifts are endless. You are an asshole.

Ash and I just laugh the day away. When life kicks you
right in the gut, you might as well find some humor in it. We
agree that one day we will look back and laugh at this particular
low point in our lives. She's just experienced an unexpected
breakup and I have cancer. Getting dumped sucks. Cancer blows.
Not the best of times...but everything is better if you can find a

way to laugh about it with a friend. We spend the next few days on the sofa binging Netflix and laughing more. She feeds my kids... keeps them laughing. She does my laundry, scrubs my toilets, and makes sure I take my meds. You can't put a price on friends like that. Ash is worth far more than gold.

Love my Ashley Farless.

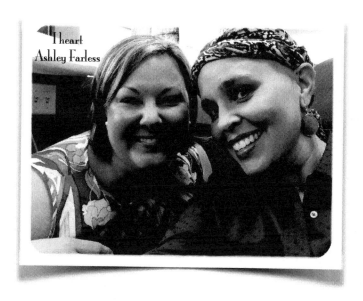

Remember that part about finding happiness and peace of mind among any circumstance? It is getting harder. I find myself annoyed as I watch others' lives proceed with perceived normalcy. I feel frustration with days seeming to fall away without anything to show. House arrest is a mounting mental challenge. I feel physically wrecked. Never has there been such a fine line between knowing how much to push my body and how much to rest.

Ordinary life seems to be pulsing all around me, and I feel disconnected and alone.

During cancer treatment, you must learn to adapt. Adapt faster and better than anyone should ever have to. Adapt to physical pain...emotional stress and fatigue...financial panic. We all have burdens to bear in life, but balancing surgeries, treatment, and life and death decisions with raising a family, an often deployed husband, and financial strain was becoming awfully heavy.

Breathe in. Breathe out. Remember that comparison is the thief of joy. Be content and grateful for the here and now. The laughter of my husband. The setting sun. The hugs and kisses from my children. The kindness of strangers. The fun I have with friends. I focus on life's sweetest moments...then I remember just how fortunate I am.

Gratitude is the ultimate gateway.

As chemo progresses, the days begin to blur more and more. My blood counts continue to suffer, though not as severely thanks to Neulasta. But—nothing comes easy. That amazing Neulasta makes my bones hurt so badly that I cry as I try to sleep at night. And I am not a crier.

Food still tastes nasty. My eyes water ALL the time. My nose bleeds. My gums bleed. My lungs burn. My body aches. I feel exhausted. There is a constant whooshing sound in my head from my anemia. I can't think straight.

I hope this shit is working.

Breathe in. Breathe out. One. More. Round.

CHEMO 4

My dear mom makes it in to help me through the last round. Though I have felt horrible for three solid weeks, by the grace of God, I actually feel decent the Sunday before my final treatment on Monday. We take in a show at the Majestic Theatre downtown. (If you are ever in San Antonio, please go. It is a beautiful venue.) Our day is filled with my favorite things: giggles, guffaws, good food, and cocktails. Boudro's on the Riverwalk. Mmmmmmmmmmmm fresh mojito for me and prickly pear margarita for mom.

Life is good.

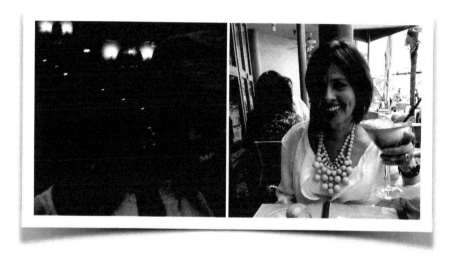

As I lay my head down to sleep that night, I do so in gratitude for the helpers. I think about how Mister Rogers said that his mother told him that we should look for helpers when we see scary things on the news, because we would always find people helping. The same is true for scary things happening front and center in our own lives; we should look for the helpers. Then we should *let them help us*. Then we should thank our lucky stars to have them.

I wake Monday filled with both excitement and dread. Thrilled to be checking off my last treatment. Fearful of just how bad the effects of the last round will be.

You know the drill…weigh in. I've gained two more pounds by eating even less than I did the previous round. Nice. (I could have guessed that the number on the scale would go up. Steroids don't do you any favors in the weight department. And, I am starting to get cankles since one of my chemo drugs damages capillaries so much that fluid leaks from them causing swelling in the legs and weight gain from fluid retention. Lovely.) IV troubles, of course. Meds. Many laughs with mom. Next-day Neulasta shot. Flu-feeling and searing bone pain. Steroid insomnia. Burning tears of frustration.

A week passes and it is time for the follow-up with my oncologist. I get an F on my blood work again...which is both bad and good. Bad because my counts have tanked and hit rock bottom again despite the Neulasta, but good in the respect that we bombarded my body with all the chemo it could tolerate. (That is if you can say that totally wiping out your immune system is a good thing. Sometimes I wonder.....) No more poison will be pumped through me. I hope I never, ever, ever have to endure chemo again. We will do a follow-up PET scan in six months. The next part of the plan will include chemically shutting down my ovaries until they can be surgically removed. I figure that my oncologist will give me a few weeks to recover, then we'll cross that bridge. Well, I thought like Lit! I will be given a bone density scan and if the results are favorable, chemical menopause will begin in ONE week.

(Recall that my tumor was fueled by and extremely, greedily hungry for both estrogen and progesterone. Ergo, I don't need any estrogen or progesterone circulating to promote growth of any cancer cells that may have survived chemo. Why the bone density scan? Estrogen plays a vital role in bone health. As estrogen declines, the incidence of osteoporosis increases...even with a healthy diet and exercise. We'll need to ensure that my bones are healthy enough to withstand the estrogen deprivation.)

The bone density scan is the easiest diagnostic test yet. No fasting. No needles. No enclosures in tiny spaces. Finally, an A+ on a test! It seems my bones are in fantastic health. Hooray for calcium and weight-bearing exercise my whole life. Looks like they did my bones good!

Since the bone density scan is good, I am a 'go' for Zoladex induced menopause. I find out that the shot is administered in the chemo treatment room. Dang! I thought I was forever done with that place! The shot is a bit of a pain, but over and done with much faster than chemo. I am given an ice pack to place on my belly for fifteen minutes, which screams to me that I am about to encounter a Boss Hog of a needle. I am right— that sucker is huge and spring-loaded. Once my skin is nice, cold, and pink, the nurse pinches my skin and asks me if I am ready. Breathe in. Breathe out. "Yes, I am ready." In the needle goes...a few inches...yikes! Then the spring is triggered and the rice-pellet sized medicine pack is inserted. This will be the drill every 28 days for almost a year until my ovaries are removed. Additionally, I am placed on an oral medicine called Femara which is an aromatase

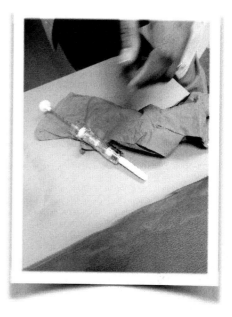

inhibitor. Aromatase from your adrenal glands takes other things in your body and converts them into small amounts of estrogen, even after menopause. So, I like to say that I am in menopause plus.

Ever thought about exactly what makes a woman a woman? I sure hope the answer is not boobs and estrogen, because now I am void of both. HOLY HOT FLASH! Instant menopause...no easing into it. Karma is laughing at me...again. I can recall so many times seeing my mom melt into a puddle as she furiously fanned herself. I would laugh and laugh and she'd quip, "Just you wait! You'll have them one day and they are so awwwwwful!". (If you didn't imagine that phrase with an Alabama accent coming from a petite, feisty lady: read the sentence once more.) I never thought we'd experience hot flashes at the same time! Ha! Now, having spent my entire life hot natured and sweaty, I THOUGHT I understood. Ashley Farless and I used to turn our dorm room into a tundra…which felt perfectly comfy to us. Others would shiver as we sighed Ahhhhhhhh. So….I expected a hot flash to feel like being really hot. Nuh-uh. Not. At. All. A hot flash is an entirely different animal. You can go from feeling completely normal and absolutely comfortable to OMG-there is a fireball in my belly and I am about to spontaneously combust but first I may pass out due to the light-headedness hot. I'd swear I was about to burst into flames. I should have never laughed at my mom!

At least now we can laugh together…

Insomnia and joint pain are the other two little gifts courtesy of Zoladex and Femara. Over time, I learn that exercise, more exercise, and essential oils help me manage these side effects to some degree.

I am now 12 days past my last chemo and I finally lug myself to the gym. My body feels destroyed. I walk so slowly on the treadmill that anyone….even a granny with a walker…could have passed me. My Pilates is performed in super slow motion, likely with poor form as well… but I am out doing it! People still stare, but I no longer care. I will my body to match the warrior spirit building inside me. It feels so wonderful to do something kind and restorative for my body.

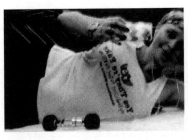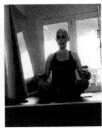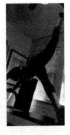

This was a turning point for me that felt like a rebirth of sorts. For a while, when I was feeling so sick, nauseated and miserable during chemo, I would grumble that it felt worse than nausea from morning sickness. And I wasn't even getting a cute baby at the end of it all...sniff, sniff.

What hit me was this: I *was* getting a new life out of the whole process.

Only this time, it was my own.

Six

Let's Rebuild

Chemo is over! My exchange surgery is just around the corner. My expanders will be removed and my permanent implants will be placed. Part of me feels like singing Ding Dong, the Witch is Dead as I envision the nasty cancer cells melllllltinggggg away and disappearing forever. The other part of me feels anxiety creeping. No longer am I pouring ammunition into my body to sweep for cancer cells. Was it enough? Did it do its job? I am acutely aware that I have never wanted to win something so badly…this battle for life. Along with anxiety, the fear of death creeps in again. (Maybe it is because, on the heels of chemo, I still feel like death.) The fear isn't ubiquitous, rather it comes and goes. I do not dwell on it, but when it sneaks in…it is painful. I know the thoughts are morbid, but I would be remiss if I led you to believe that they never crossed my mind. With the fear of dying come thoughts like: I wonder if anyone would know that Sarah Jayne smelled sweet like maple syrup when she was born. Would anyone realize that I thought she looked as if she'd be sprinkled with fairy dust when she was an infant and that Ashley Farless changed her first diaper? Would they know that when she said her feet were fizzy it meant that they were asleep? Would they recall how it felt when Maggie began to call me Mom instead of Miss Natalie? Who would be aware that when Genevieve said that her eyebrows hurt it meant that she had a headache. The only person who would remember that she was lulled to sleep by Norah Jones when she was only 24 hours old would be David. My David. Who would love him like I do? The thoughts were so overwhelming. Crippling. So when they would bubble up, I would quickly send them away. It would take time before I learned how to better manage those fears.

David arrives home in time for my exchange surgery. The five months the expanders have been in place feel much longer. The expanders are incredibly uncomfortable, and they look absolutely bizarre. They sit high on my chest - just below my collarbones - not where real boobs would ever be. My plastic surgeon assures me that my forever foobs will not rest in the same place. Thank God. I really don't care to hide under a muumuu for the rest of my life.

The surgery is much shorter than the bilateral mastectomy, lasting only a few hours. The scars from my mastectomy are opened…flesh and muscle sliced through again. The expanders are removed and replaced with saline implants. OH! Good news: This time around, I am not sedated with Propofol. I am given a different cocktail in an attempt to cut down on the post-op nausea. BINGO! Though it is harder to wake after surgery, having my nausea better under control is so worth it. *Not* vomiting with a stitched-up chest makes me want to put on my, my, my, my boogie shoes. What a relief!

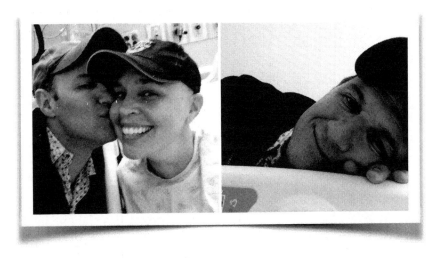

I have drains again. Only two this time…one on each side. I figure they'll be there a week since this surgery was less physically traumatic than the bilateral mastectomy.

David and I head home the next day. He will be home only a week or so, then he will have to return to Afghanistan until July. The twice daily drill of cleaning, emptying, and measuring the output of the drains resumes. We are pros at it now. This round, the drains are proving to be a bit more of a pain than last time. The output is looking more clear, but the volume refuses to decrease. The drains cannot be removed until the volume reaches a certain level. I attribute the excess fluid to the fact that my post-chemo/ node-dissection body is simply slow to recover. Makes sense to me. Plus—one of the drain tubes seems to be rubbing against a nerve. There is a constant burning sensation…and when it moves a certain way….HOLY HELL! It hurts so badly that I wince and gasp for air. I've got this, though. Breathe in. Breath out.

Surely these suckers will be out soon.

Foiled again. It is time for David to re-deploy, and I still have both drains. Awesome. Fun times.

Not long after David leaves, my sweet friend Kate arrives. She comes at the perfect time. Her hugs and laughs are just what the doctor ordered. She is a huge help in so many ways….especially with packing up my house. (Did I mention we are moving in a few weeks? Only a mile away, but the house must be packed nonetheless.)

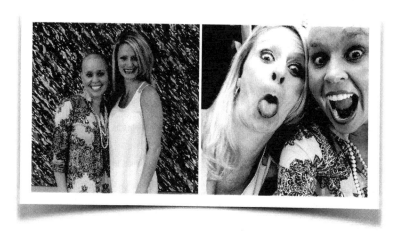

While she is there, I am walking past some boxes and one of the tubes to my drain snags the edge. Ouch! Uh-oh. The drains have been in several weeks, and I guess I have grown too accustomed to them. The tubes are usually tucked under my shirt, but one of them had somehow worked its way out and found that edge of a box. I go to take a look, and the stitches have been torn from my body. The end of the drain tube is still inside of me, but it has definitely moved. Of course, it is Saturday. Do unfortunate slip-ups, accidents, sick kids, or any other miserable semi-emergency events ever happen any time other than the weekend or after business hours?

I get in touch with the on-call plastics doctor at MDA. He asks me if the bulb is still holding suction. Yes? Ok— that is good. That means the end of the drain tube is still in the capsule of muscle where it needs to be. The part that has slid out cannot be pushed back in since that would be a sure way to push bacteria into my body. The doctor says that he will meet me at the ER at MDA (3 hrs away) to repair the damage. However, he lets me know that it is highly likely that a tiny slip of the tube will be too much and that the bulb will lose suction. After more discussion, we decide that instead of making the six hour round trip drive to Houston, I should go to a local ER and have stitches placed to keep the tube from moving.

Sweet Kate takes over with my girls, taking the best care and entertaining them while I wheel myself to the ER.

I arrive at the ER where I am quickly seen. I have to explain the whole situation. The triage nurse finds it hard to believe that I am a cancer patient being as I am relatively young and since I look "fit". The doctor shares the same sentiment. Guess what…cancer doesn't discriminate, friends. I have to explain that the tube can't be pushed back in, but it can be stitched to hold its place. The doctor carefully stitches the tube so that it will hold. I sign some papers, and I am on my way.

Would you believe that five minutes….FIVE MINUTES… into my drive home————I hear whooooooooooosh.

The bulb has lost suction.

Really? Seriously? Yep. Arrrrrgggghhhhhh.

Now the tube must be removed. I do not want to spend any more time the in ER, so my nurse friend Carole comes to my house and removes both my stitches and the drain. The village is stepping in to come to my aid, again. I have been the recipient of so many kind gestures, every one of which I will be forever grateful.

I have a pep talk with my body. "Puhhhhhhhleazzzze. Pretty, pretty please pick up the slack for that drain and absorb this excess fluid. You've got this, body. I know you can do it. I beeeeeelieve in you."

Alas, my pep talk is a bust.

The next day, my right foob is enormous and red. Looks like I will be hitting the road for MDA after all. I make the the 3 hour trek to MDA. With one look the doctor lets me know that yep, I am going to need a new drain. Of course I will. And of course it is late afternoon which means there is neither an available operating room nor an available Interventional Radiologist to see me that day. Yes, of course. I scramble to arrange a hotel room for the night and for my sweet friend Kate to spend another night with my girls.

Since I drove myself to Houston and I don't want to spend yet *another* night there, I plead with my surgeon and the IR doctor agree to let me have the procedure with local anesthesia. Gratefully, they acquiesce. They give me an IV anyway (y'all know this is my favorite thing in the world) just in case they need it. Into my couture hospital gown I go. (Why are hospital gowns so ugly??) This will be the first time that I am wide awake and fully aware of my surroundings in the operating room. I actually find it pretty fascinating. The IR doc talks me through the entire procedure. He numbs me, makes a small incision, and uses a big contraption to guide the drain tube into the right spot in my chest wall. The drain is placed with no problems, and he stitches me up. I hang out in recovery for a bit and then get dressed and hit the road for San Antonio.

Home sweet home.

Another week passes, and it is time to head to Atlanta for the wedding of Sarah Jayne's aunt Rachel. Sarah Jayne will be the flower girl, and we have been looking forward to it for months. I still have both drains....blah. Maybe it isn't the best time to hop on a plane with two kids, but we are going anyway. Why not just skip it? Cancer has already sidelined me too many times this year. I want to go to the wedding...witness bubbly love...eat, drink, and be merry....see some of our favorite people in the whole wide world, including my former Mother in Law (no joke here...she is truly one of my favorite people in the world.....and for the record, my current MIL is one of the sweetest people on the planet...I got so lucky, y'all)...laugh....LIVE.

We make it to Atlanta just fine. I have been keeping close watch on the output of my drains, and the morning of the wedding I am able to remove my left drain. Woohooo! I came prepared with a suture removal kit just in case. I have seen it done enough times that I feel confident that I can do it myself. It has been 30 days already, and I don't care to spend one extra minute with that sucker. One drain will surely be better than two. I clean the area and sterilize the scissors. I clip and pull the stitches. I breathe in. I breathe out and pull the tube from my body. Whew!

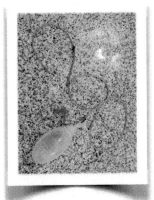

Glad that is finished. I bandage the area and get on with the fun of the day.

I can't wear the hot pink dress I had planned, because there is no way it can hide my remaining drain. Instead, I don my trusty (long) little black dress because it conceals my remaining drain. The dress may be boring black, but I complete it with some fierce boots and sparkly green earrings. My earrings are compliments of my dear Ashley Farless, gifted to me about the same time I read the book "Sparkly Green Earrings" by Melanie Shankle. I want to be like the earrings as she describes them in the book.... "Shiny, happy, and colorful, with a blinding glimmer every time they catch the light. ... Daniel 12:3 says that those who are wise will 'shine like the brightness of the heavens, and those who lead many to righteousness, like the stars for ever and ever.'"

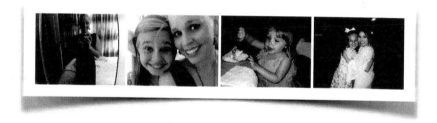

The wedding is incredibly beautiful and sweet. The bride is breathtaking. It is a blessing to witness Rachel and Travis tie the knot. The night is filled with love, laughter, dancing, delicious food, and time with people precious to us.

I savor every minute.

The time arrives to go home. We head to the airport, return the rental car, and check in. You know, we are all accustomed to the comforts of whatever bubble reside…but take yourself to the airport, and you will be quickly reminded of what a motley crew of people share our existence. I could sit and people watch at the airport for hours and not get bored. There is so much good in humanity, but I find that air travel tends to bring out very bad behavior in people. Take the time I asked a flight attendant for a little help getting my bag into the overhead bin. She promptly told me that if it was too heavy for me that it would certainly be too heavy for her. I was dumbfounded, but somehow managed to stammer that it wasn't that it was *that* heavy, it was that I was seven months *pregnant* and I had a *hernia*…In the middle of my explanation, a kind passenger stepped in and came to my rescue. Thank you, sir, for restoring my faith in humanity. Then there was the time I was totally hollow-eyed and chemo-bald at a crowded gate…sitting on the floor with two kids…as I stared at a row of people tapping away on their laptops…not a single one pausing to even offer their seat. I likely would have declined, but the offer would have been nice. Aaaaaand then there is today….while checking our bags the desk attendant says, "So, what made you shave your head like that?" My reply…. "Ummmmm. That'd be cancer, ma'am. Most expensive hairstyle I've ever had." She answers with a flat "Oh. My mom had cancer. She died."

Planes, trains, and automobiles….the struggle!

You just have to laugh.

Seven

Cry Me a River

June 2013

May turns to June.

Somewhere in there we move houses…while David is still in Afghanistan…the memory is a blur. I still have a damn drain. I feel terribly tired…both physically and mentally. I develop an infection in my right reconstructed breast. I wake one morning to find it red and swollen. And I have a fever. Not good. Back to MDA I go. I have a seroma (collection of fluid) in the pocket where my implant resides. It will need to be surgically drained. I hit the operating room another time for a drain replacement. Once again, I lobby for local anesthesia only since Genevieve is with me this time. (In the daycare, of course.) The fluid is sent for review, which reveals a host of nasty bugs that will require a barrage of antibiotics for treatment. My plastic surgeon explains that it may be rather difficult to to kick the infection especially if a biofilm has formed around the implant. He says that my chance of beating the infection is slim and that I will likely need to have the implant removed. My foes this time are: *Peptostreptococcus prevoti, Leclercia adecarboxylata, Stenotrophomonas maltophili,* and *Enterococci.* They even sound nasty, right? Please, please, please…let me kick their asses to the curb. At least my friend Lee Ann makes me laugh by saying I may soon earn the moniker "The Uniboober".

The three antibiotics that I am given are brutal. They are "black box" drugs, and they cause some major reactions. Insomnia. Vertigo. Vomiting. (These particular ones can also cause spontaneous rupture of connective tissues.) The vertigo is so bad that it is really difficult to manage myself, much less take care of children. There is a substitute for one of them and once we make that change, things are somewhat better. I am able to sleep a little more. The vertigo lessens to just general dizziness. I am nauseous, but not vomiting. I have to take the meds twice a day. I learn that if I choke them down, get horizontal and take to the sofa or bed for an hour, I can keep the pills from coming back up. So I do that in the morning and again in the evening.

Sarah Jayne is in Alabama for the next several weeks. It is just me and little Genevieve....and a lot of TV. (Actually it is a lot of streaming video on the computer. I am not attempting to set up the TV in the new house.) Our current BFFs are Bubble Guppies. Octonauts. Mickey Mouse Clubhouse. Max and Ruby. Max and his incredibly annoying, bossy, whiney, sister Ruby.

David is still deployed. With all of my insomnia, I have come to appreciate his erratic sleep patterns. When he is home, I have someone to hang out with when insomnia strikes. Now, I reach in the darkness and do not find him, making me acutely aware of his absence.

I am not really a big crier, but June brings river of tears. I think I actually cry at least once a day for the whole month. It seems that EVERYTHING makes me cry. The good and the bad. I still have a drain....waaaaah. I am so tired....waaaah waaaaah. There are harsh phantom pains where my breasts used to be... boohoo. The sunset is gorgeous....boohooohoooooo. I miss David.... sobbbbbbbb. Genevieve says something incredibly sweet....sniffsniffsniff. I open the door and the muddy dog runs through the house.....waaaiiiiiillll. Ridiculous, I know. I take inventory of the fact that I am alive and breathing, and you guessed it, I cry more. Happy tears, but tears nonetheless.

Since diagnosis, I have been in battle mode. Staying strong for each and every round of the fight has been necessary. Now that things are slowing a bit, there is time to process some of the buried emotions. Cue the tears. I also assumed that things would be so much easier when chemo was over....that cancer would basically be done. So many times I had thought to myself, "Just make it through chemo. It will all be downhill after that. It will be breezy. Just hang on.". The reality is....things are still hard. I feel kicked in the gut by this new infection. I feel broken.

I have had the remaining drain for an eternity. I am going to have to dream up some sort of alternative use for it....punishing the kids maybe. "If you don't straighten up and act right, it is your turn to clean the drain!"

But...I breathe in. I breathe out. I push forward.

I allow the negative emotions leave my body with the tears that fall. I focus thoughts and energy on Romans 8:28 "We know that all things work together for good for those who love God, who are called according to his purpose." I choose to surrender my brokenness and let good take its place.

In other news, I am starting to get a bit of fuzz on my head...hoooray! It comes with a price, though. I also have very soft, fine, peach fuzz hair all over my face. Just like newborn babies have. Monkey face. Could be worse....at least they are not whiskers!

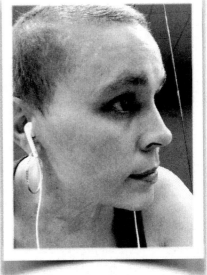

As June comes to an end, things are looking up.

The infection seems to be clearing. After 60 days...yes, I said sixty... the drain is finally removed. It looks like I won't have to be The Uniboober after all, whew!

Also, David returns home! Ahhhhhhhh. A reprieve.

Shelter from the storm.

Eight

Sweet Relief

July and August 2013

Sweet relief. No more drains. No surgeries this month or next. My family is back together. The chemo fog is beginning to fade. My hair is growing! What started as a few sprouts in June actually resembles a short and edgy style now. My chemo bloat and swelling is getting much better. I am feeling my energy build….somewhat. Life is good.

I am beginning to understand that for those who've had to fight hard for it, life has a flavor that the protected may never fully know. I am aware of all the blessings in my life, and I see them with incredible clarity. I do not know anyone whose life has played out as planned, but I do know that the happiest are those who keep living, learning, creating. Who keep chasing new dreams. Who keep filling the pages in their rich book of life.

Do not wait for someone to give you permission to live. You don't have to wait for things to feel perfectly aligned to move forward…..one of the many lessons taught to me by cancer. It is absolutely your birthright to dive right in and make the most of your fabulous life.

July brings me to my six-month post-mastectomy checkup with my breast surgeon. There is a certain security in tooling around MDA. These are my people. No one looks twice or stares at bald heads. Head scarves. Fuzzy heads. Monkey-hair faces. Chemo curls. Missing appendages. Swollen faces or limbs. Bandages. Hospital ID bands. Ports. Scars. IV poles. Many nationalities are represented and multiple languages are spoken. There are men and women. Young adults. Kids. Old people. Everything in between. And every single person there has cancer in common. Either they are the patient….or they are supporting the patient or they are treating the patient. There is no awkwardness. A certain kinship exists, and it is easy to strike up conversation with most anyone. For this, I am grateful.

"Could a greater miracle take place than for us to look through each other's eyes for an instant?"
Henry David Thoreau

When crossing one of the MDA sky bridges, there is an adjacent building in view with tiles down the side forming images of strands of DNA. Every time I see it, I am left wondering how something so nebulous as a tiny DNA mutation can manifest into something as giant, real, and threatening as cancer? I used to teach both Biology and Chemistry, so of course I understand the mechanics of it…but still….it blows my mind that something so microscopically tiny can have such far-reaching influences that can ultimately result in death. Yikes.

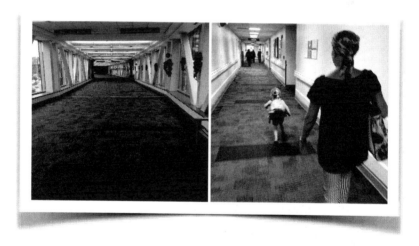

The meeting with my breast surgeon goes well. My foobies are coming along nicely, but there is a palpable lymph node in my right axillary region that warrants further testing. I hadn't really felt it. Well actually I had, but I couldn't distinguish it from the multitude of other lumps and bumps of scar tissue in the same area. The node is biopsied, and thankfully, all is clear!

We also meet with my plastic surgeon to discuss my next reconstructive surgery. It will include fat grafting to fill in some of the indentations around the implants. In the same surgery, a cut will be made around my nipples and they will be repositioned. The ports will be removed from the implants. The surgery will take place in September.

My new boobs are as hard as can be. We discuss options. There is a chance that they will soften over time. My surgeon explains that we can wait and see or he can perform a capsulotomy. A capsulotomy involves making a network of incisions across the muscles of my chest to release the tissue that has severely tightened. Since there is a chance that the muscles will release on their own, and since a capsulotomy would definitely require more drains, I opt for the "wait and see" approach.

It is now the end of July, so that leaves some time in early August for a little fun, family time, and back-to-school activities for the girls.

The heavens part, and a week opens up with no doctor appointments for me…no dentist appointments for anyone in the family…no school or sports activities for any of the kids. As soon as we realize we have this gift of time, we pack up and get out of town. Beach, here we come! The five of us road-trip it to Orange Beach, AL. Ahhhhhhhhh. I have always LOVED having my toes in the sand, and this trip is no different. I delight in relaxing and laughing with David, in watching my girls play, and in spending time with my mom and dad.

We get the idea to try parasailing. I have always wanted to try it, and now it feels like there is no time like the present. I am done with putting things off.

We decide David will go up with Maggie and Sarah Jayne. He has jumped from a million planes and helicopters, so this is no biggie for him. His relaxed attitude keeps the girls calm and light-hearted. Up, up, and away they go! The smiles on their faces fill me with glee and a deep, deep contentment. The boat captain reels them in and it is time for mom and for me. I am a little nervous, but I can't let it show now…my eleven and thirteen year old daughters just tackled it with no fear!

As we head up, the butterflies in my stomach disappear. It is so very peaceful. Why haven't I done this before??? Cheesy as it may sound, I feel triumphant. I could dangle up here all day long. It is such a welcome, quiet escape from all the noise surrounding me every day. For a moment or two, no thoughts are present in my head....only

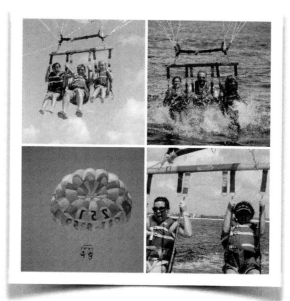

peacefulness and awe at the beauty of the world. Serenity.

Our vacation comes to a close, and we head back to San Antonio. We ready the girls for school. Maggie will be in the eighth grade. Sarah Jayne will be in sixth....her debut to Junior School. Genevieve will be in preschool for the first time. Call me a huge nerd, but I have always liked the back-to-school time. A new year full of possibilities...new faces....new experiences. A time for growth. (Rosy as I am painting it at the moment, we all know that the grind is felt after a while....Is it really time to rise in the dark? Again? You need whaaaaaat for a project? By tomorrow? You lost your lunchbox.....again?)

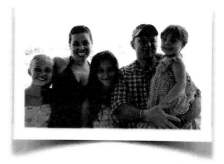

At any rate, I appreciate the freshness of new potential.

Nine

Tune up

September 2013

The school year is off to a good start. With David home and a break from surgeries, I have had a chance to catch my breath.

Just in time for my next surgery.

Breathe in. Breathe out. Here we go.

Again.

David has to be in South Korea for a short bit, so my mom is coming to MDA with me. The kids will be staying with sweet Louisa.

Mom is my buddy as we do the pre-op day shuffle. Meetings with the plastic surgeon. Labs. Surgery scheduler, etc. MDA....Most of the Day Anderson. We make the most of it and find lots of laughter. The laughs started the night before as we parked the car at the Rotary House. I am behind the wheel when we pull up to valet parking. As we exit the car, the attendant directs his attention to me and asks me if my mom will be needing any assistance. I tell him, "No, no....she is okay". The he asks for her name and her MRN, to which I reply, "Her last name is Davis, but she doesn't have a Medical Record Number. However, my last name is Holland and my MRN is ......" I suppose I must be looking pretty healthy! On the other hand, mom must need a nap and to freshen her makeup. Ha!

We are staying at the Rotary House, so it is easy to walk downstairs to enjoy a cocktail at the hotel restaurant. Again, it is easy to feel relaxed alongside my cancer cohorts. Looking around, the people there are obviously in various states of health. Some are new to the MDA shuffle...some are there for checkups...some are there for surgeries...some are there for treatment. The crowd is full of bald heads and hospital ID bands. There is even a man hooked up to his IV pole enjoying an ice cold beer. Cheers

Everyone there is moving forward. Enjoying life. Still smiling. Still laughing. Still appreciating every breath drawn.

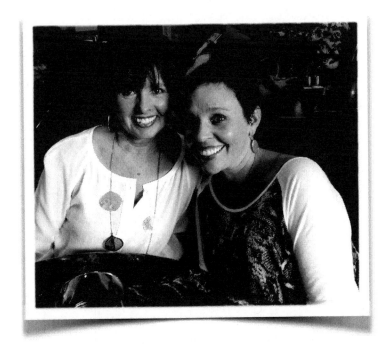

The next day begins like all other surgery days.....no food....no makeup....no jewelry. I am asked the same questions again and again in pre-op to ensure that everyone is on the same page. Propophol will not be used...thank God!

I am wheeled into the operating room. I drift into my long nap. All goes well. Again, it is *so very difficult* to wake after surgery, but worth avoiding nausea and vomiting.

I sleep most of the day. I am bruised, sore and stitched, but the pain is minor compared to the previous major surgeries. Just what did they do this time? Well, breast tissue extends above your actual boobs to your upper chest area. Every bit of that tissue was removed in my bilateral mastectomy. This left some pretty serious divots above my foobs. If I lift my arms, big concave indentations form across my chest. In an effort to help fill the holes and make the transition from my chest area to my breast area more natural, fat was grafted from my belly and transplanted to my chest area. Also, a portion of the old scars on each breast was opened and the ports were removed from my implants. Finally, since my nipples had shifted around during the healing process, they had to be tweaked. To accomplish this, incisions were made around the nipples, some skin was excised, and then they were sewn back in place. They will be given time to heal and settle, then the process will be repeated.

Once again, my chest looks like Frankenstein. I am not really bothered by it, though. Rather, I feel fascinated that skilled surgeons can build boobs....out of nothing. (Cue the Air Supply....Making boobs....out of nothing at all...making boooooooobs, outta nothing at all.)

Mom and I spend the night in Houston and head back to San Antonio the next day. The kids are happy to have us back, and I find myself feeling thankful that my mom has been able to spend so much time with us. She will stay one more night then leave early the next morning. David will fly in late afternoon. Yes, our house is often like a revolving door.

David is home for a few more days, then it is time for him to go. Again. Sigggghhhhhh. Time for a little more of that absence that makes the heart grow fonder. I do not know where I would be without him. His hugs warm my heart and soothe my soul. His gaze still makes me melt, and his touch heals my broken spirit.

The next week I take part in a fashion show benefitting the American Cancer Society. My gorgeous friend Michelle is in charge of the show, and she invites me to model. So much fun! I get a makeover....I get free cocktails....and I get to wear fabulous clothes and strut down the runway. No doubt something my five foot three self never thought I would do! The cast is a mix of cancer survivors and some professional models. The cancer bunch is a ton of fun....warm....full of laughs. It feels amazing to do something fun to benefit the ACS, which has been paramount in helping me navigate the complex load of information that comes with cancer.

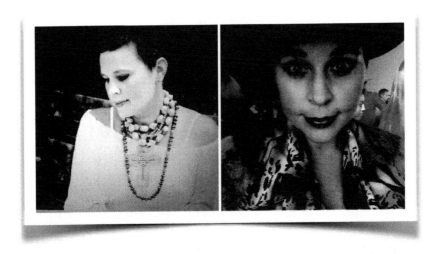

It is good that I've had something fun on which to focus since my six month post-chemo checkup is right around the corner. I will have a PET scan and then meet with my oncologist a week later. I would be fibbing if I said I wasn't nervous. I am feeling well, but cancer is stealth like that…it snuck up the first time around. Who is to say that it isn't back?

Here we go again. I fast the night before, and arrive to the START center with a growling tummy. An IV is started, and it delivers the radioactive sugar molecules to my bloodstream. Mmmmmmmmmm…..radioactive sugar. I am reminded not to hug or hold my kids for the remainder of the day. I flip through some magazines as I wait the hour for the marked molecules to circulate through my body. I feel pretty peaceful. At this point, I know that it is what it is. Being a nervous ball-o-stress won't help me anyway. Keep Calm and Fight On.

The actual scan is much like before….easy. I have learned to just close my eyes and breathe deeply so that being enclosed in such a small space doesn't panic me. I doze for a few minutes, then the test is finished. I know the techs can tell a lot by the images they have just seen. I also know that they cannot tell me a thing. A week I will have to wait. When awaiting test results, it seems you feel time differently. The days pass so slowly.

Finally, it is Monday. My precious friend Fawn is going with me since David is away. Fun Fawn is an amazing friend....accompanying me to Houston for expander fills.....listening patiently to all of my cancer woes....celebrating little victories with me.....and LAUGHING with me. Though we haven't been friends for a long time, we just click....no surprise since we are birthday twins! Has the universe sent me some gems or what?

Fawn's presence calms me as we wait for my doctor to enter the room. In he comes.....I am all smiles and belt out, "Tell me something good!". He responds with, "Wellllllllllll.........".

Oh.

Well.

Shit. Shitshitshitshit. My stomach does a flip and sinks. For a brief moment, I feel as if I am caught in that same tunnel I found myself trapped in the day I was first diagnosed. The air feels thinner and it is hard to breathe or hear what anyone is saying. Ok, Natalie. Breathe in. Breathe out. Snap into focus. We get right to the business of discussing what is up. He explains that a node in my right axillary region lit up the PET scan. We do chat about the fact that it has only been three weeks since my last surgery and that it could possibly be reactionary to that. The only way to know for sure would be another biopsy, which will be performed the same day.

First I have to head down one floor to get my monthly Zoladex shot. The nurses in the chemo treatment room are always cheerful and nice....it is the front desk crew that could use a crash course in social pleasantries. As I check in, to ensure records are up to date, I am asked a few questions.

This is how the conversation goes:

Front desk dude: Are you still at blahblahblah address with yadayadayada insurance carrier?

Me: Yes, that is correct.

Dude: And your employment status….with an eyebrow raise… *stilllll unemployed*???

Me: That's right.
Dude (crinkling his nose and furrowing his brow): You mean you don't work at allllll?

Me: Nope.

What I wish I had said:

Well, there exists the small matters of cancer, chemo, multiple surgeries, infections and hospitalizations…then you have my preteens, my toddler, the dog and the fish all to care for while my husband is overseas….oh, and yes, I am actively pursuing Pilates certification…taking classes and working on hours….Oh, and my new hair. Well, my Bob Ross Afro, also known as my Justin Timberfro, takes so much time to tame that it is practically a job all of its own…. So, maybe I should say that
YES, I WORK…..FOR FREE.

Have a nice day *ya giant butthole*.

So many times I have wished for the gift of the snappy comeback. Alas, I always think of a quip hours….or days later.

Sweet Fawn stays with me - putting off her need to return to work. Girlfriends are the best. I get the Zoladex rice pellet shot into my belly, then we head down one more floor to check in for the biopsy. More needles. Marvelous. An ultrasound guides the radiologist to the suspicious node. He pulls the needed fluid, and I am on my way.

I feel disappointed, but hopeful that it is nothing at all. Fawn keeps me laughing. It occurs to me that cancer has made me stronger. More resilient. The same news a year ago would have reduced me to a teary mess. Ohblahdee, Ohblahda, life goes on….lalalalala life goes on….

I make it home in time to help with homework, fix dinner, and tame a toddler. After the girls are in bed, I busy myself with removing the sutures from my latest surgery. I clip and pull stitches from my nipples, my port holes, and my fat-grafting site.

As I drift to sleep, my prayer is that the results will come swiftly.

Jen

Those Sweet Words

October 2013

It's Pinktober, y'all.

I mean it is October 1st. It has been almost a year since my diagnosis on the 24th of last October. Still unsure if I am showing no evidence of disease, I am anxiously awaiting that call from my nurse.

Thankfully, I do not have to wait long…the call comes in the afternoon. The results are in, and I am CANCER FREE!!!! Did you hear that?!?!?!?! CANCER FREEEEEEEEEEEEEE!!!!!! Tears of joy stream down my face. I feel a special sort of jubilation. Glee. Relief. Though it is a different kind of emotion, the intensity ranks right up there with the birth of my babies.

October 1st, 2013 happens to be a school night, so there isn't much time for a formal celebration. I spend some time letting David and all the people I love know that the news is great. Fawn shows up with a bottle of wine and we celebrate with sushi, laughs, and dances with my girls.

I wake on Wednesday, October 2 with an enormous smile on my face. However, I feel a bit off. I wake Sarah Jayne for school and cook her breakfast. Hmmmm. I really do not feel well. At this point, I am sure you are suspecting a big ole hangover to be the culprit, but I only indulged in two glasses of wine. Surely it cannot be a hangover. I scratch an itch just above my foob. It looks a little red. Hmmmmm. Maybe it is because I just scratched there. That's gotta be it. I make a point not to touch it again, and I am certain the redness will fade. I see Sarah Jayne off to walk to school. Since Genevieve seems to be sleeping late, I crawl back in bed to try to sleep an extra hour to rid myself of this funky feeling. When I awake around an hour later, I've gone from feeling bad to feeling absolutely lousy. The small red spot has grown, and it is now warm to the touch. I have a 102 degree fever accompanied by chills.

I immediately call my plastic surgeon, who phones in two antibiotics. Things have escalated quickly. By now, I am too weak to even drive. My sweet friend Heather picks up my meds. I feel awful and too sick to do anything the remainder of the day. Thank God for my Sarah Jayne who knows how to order delivery and give her sister a bath. I stay in the bed the rest of the evening. I intermittently check on the girls and they do the same for me. I wake the next day, and though my fever has improved slightly, the redness is worse and has spread. My chest is swollen, red, and hot to the touch. David tells me to mark the red area on my skin with a Sharpie so I can better monitor the progress. (He never gets his feathers ruffled under pressure…always just calmly makes recommendations for what the next move should be.) I take another round of antibiotics in hopes of vast improvement. My fever is still hovering. The redness continues to spread. My surgeon calls to check on me and tells me that I need to come to Houston to MDA to be seen. He tells me that I will likely need IV antibiotics. I scramble around and find a friend to watch Genevieve. She assures me that both Genevieve and Sarah Jayne can stay with her for the night if my babysitter is unable to stay. I pack an overnight bag, drop Genevieve at her house and hit the road to Houston. I get in touch with Saint Louisa, and she lets me know she can take care of the girls for the night.

By some miracle, I make it to MDA late that afternoon. I have no idea how I really made the drive. I am seen by the on-call doctor in the reconstructive surgery center. I do not recall his exact words, but they basically conveyed, "This is bad". He lets me know that I definitely need to be admitted for IV antibiotics. Just as I was mentally congratulating myself for having the foresight to pack an overnight bag…he adds that I will be in the hospital for a minimum of five to seven days. Whaaaaaaaaaaaat? I do not know whether to laugh or cry. Who is going to watch my kids? How am I going to survive a week with one spare pair of undies? Oh dear.

I immediately call my mama. At first she can't really make out what I am saying, because I am in fact, half laughing and half crying. I am sure I sound like a crazed lunatic. Ok. Breathe in. Breathe out. I slow down and explain my predicament. She tells me she is going to hang up so she can figure out how soon she can hop on a plane.

I walk myself and my admission papers to the admissions office of the hospital. After a bit of waiting, they get me checked in and tell me where to report. When I arrive on my floor of the infectious disease wing, the nurses are in the middle of a shift change. I ask to be directed to the room number I was assigned. Amidst the shuffle, someone points me in the right direction. I plop down in the chair next to the bed. I. Am. Exhausted. Some time passes and a nurse finally arrives and asks me where the patient is. I laugh and tell her that I *am* the patient. She laughs, apologizes, and lets me know that she thought I was visiting someone. Just another example that we never really know the battles others may be fighting. In my "street clothes", I look pretty normal since I am no longer bald. (Now that I think of it, maybe my awful hairstyle should have been a hint. I should have never had ill thoughts about that surgeon who looked like Gene Wilder, because I am now his twin in the hair department. Yikes! Karma.) One peek under my shirt or a look at my blood work would def give away my secret. I don my hospital gown. Of course, it is ugly. A sweet nurse comes in and starts my IV...y'all know how much I lovvvvvvve needles and IVs. Thankfully, he is very good. He flushes my line, and my mouth fills with the taste of rubbing alcohol. Blechhhhh.

Now, I am just waiting for the treatment plan. It is quiet save for the drip of the IV, the whoosh of the air in the hospital bed, and the loud growl of my stomach. Sigh. Alone with my thoughts. I really miss my girls. There are surely times that I'd love to duct tape them to the wall just so I could have a moment of peace, but in this moment, I would love nothing more than to scoop them up...hug them tightly...feel their soft cheeks brush across my face....and hear them say I love you. I also miss David terribly. At least there is FaceTime....

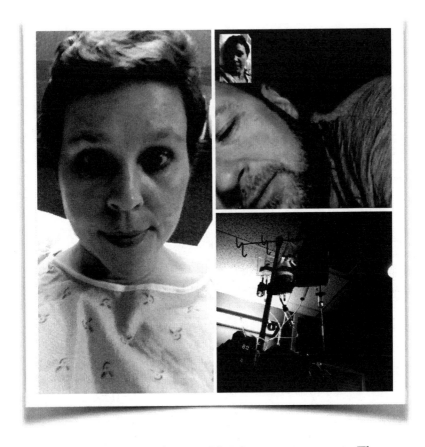

Another nurse arrives and begins my treatment. Three different IV antibiotics. One of them burns like crazy as it enters my veins so they slow the drip hoping I can better tolerate it. Another will make me pee bright orange for days.

My phone rings, and it is my mom. She tells me that she and my dad have booked the first flights out in the morning. My dad will stop in Houston and grab a cab to MDA, and my mom will continue to San Antonio. Love. That's what that is. Frankie and Jayne may not be the most verbal when it comes to shows of affection, but their actions show their love in the biggest ways. Better to do it well than speak it well I say.

Dad arrives. We end up having a lot of laughs over the next few days while confined to an itty bitty hospital room. The one-on-one father daughter time is absolutely a silver lining to this whole debacle. I have a video of him wrestling with the chair that turns into a 'bed'. Makes me laugh so hard that is difficult to breathe! I should put it on Vine or something. Only I don't have a Vine account. I also get a visit from Charmoin, my friend from both high school and college, who happens to live in Houston. I love how the stars align to bring happy events even in the midst of crummy times.

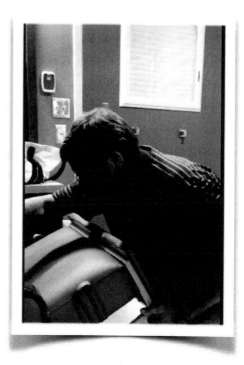

I am usually a very nice patient, and I am typically non-confrontational in any and every situation. However, Dad (who has no problem with confrontation) got to sit back and witness me have a come-apart followed by a come-to-Jesus with one of my nurses. I had great nurses that visit....except for one: Grumpy Gwen. She was grumpy and mean. I won't get into the particulars, but she just pushed my buttons one too many times and I let loose!

Nurses, listen, I know y'all have an incredibly challenging job. You have to juggle a multitude of tasks at once. I get that. BUT, bedside manner is every bit as important as your smarts. If you reach a point when you can't be patient and kind with the patients....get yourself a new job. And for all of you wonderful nurses out there, a big THANK YOU. You make a huge difference in the lives of those receiving your care.

The good news is that the infection is responding to the antibiotics. The bad news: they are so strong that they burn through and collapse a vein a day…..and man-o-man, when that happens…ouch…which means I get a new IV line every day. Since I cannot have an IV in my right arm, the daily treat of a new IV line involves lots of digging around my left arm to find a suitable vein. Groovy.

Five days later, I spring the joint. I am given three strong oral antibiotics which thankfully allows me to avoid going home with a PICC (peripherally inserted central catheter) line. The antibiotics are merciless on my stomach. The next two weeks are spent carefully spacing them so that they do not come right back up. Wake. Get Sarah Jayne off to school. Give Genevieve breakfast. Take one antibiotic. Get horizontal for an hour. Up again. Eat. Take two more antibiotics. Plow through the day's events. Take antibiotics and anti-nausea meds and face plant into bed. October 2013 passes pretty much like the past year has….in a haze.

October, as we all know thanks to the explosion of pink ribbons, is Breast Cancer Awareness month. As grateful as I am for awareness campaigns, sometimes I fear that the pink ribbon has become so ubiquitous, that people are unaware of all it actually represents. Even worse, some companies capitalize on it, splashing a pink ribbon on all of their products in an effort to to sell even more junk….much of which is manufactured in a manner that contributes to a host of health problems, breast cancer included. Some such companies donate little or nothing to programs that support breast cancer screening or treatment. So, please think before you pink! Remember that breast cancer is not pretty like a pink ribbon. It is needles. Bruises. Vomit. Radiation burns. Surgeries. Scars. Drains. Burning eyes and lungs from chemo. Chemo brain. Mouth sores. Nose sores. Throat sores. More scars. Hot flashes. Neutropenia. Anemia. Joint pain.

Neuropathy. Muscle stiffness. Bald heads. Chemo curls. Missing events. FOMO. Missing body parts. Missing fingernails and/or toenails. Vision and hearing changes. Rashes. And more.

Physically, I am forever changed. I can never again be a blood donor. I will never have the sensation of breasts again. I can never have blood pressure measured or blood drawn from my right arm. I have decreasing bone density from being in menopause plus at age 37. I experience a host of side effects from my maintenance medication.

But, bruises make for better conversation...right?

Tomorrow, October 24, marks my one year Cancerversary. It is late, and I am relaxing a bit with Genevieve before bedtime. As she rests her head on my chest, she wiggles and finds it difficult to find a comfortable spot. Two hard mounds take the place of that which used to be a soft place for my babies to rest their heads. The moment is at first bittersweet. Then a sense of overwhelming gratitude washes over me. I am here. I am alive. I am blessed. I am happy.

I choose to let the bitterness go. I choose the sweetness.

Cancer will test you and push you beyond your conceived limits. At the end of the day, you still have the ability to choose how you feel. You can choose how you let cancer reshape you. Cancer has left me forever changed...physically, mentally, and spiritually. It passed through me and made its mark, but I won't let it define me. I choose to let myself be changed into something better. Someone more empathetic. More loving. Someone who wants to always chase dreams.

Cancer has been the biggest struggle in my life thus far. It is said that out of our biggest struggles come our greatest discoveries. For me, I found that despite what season it is in my life, there is that endless summer inside of me...one that allows me to see the bright side of things. We will all have obstacles to overcome in life, but that is life. Beautiful, messy, full-ofsurprises, amazing, miraculous life. When we commit to chasing those dreams, we prove ourselves worthy of that miracle. Let go of the fear of the unknown, and get busy chasing your dreams. Take one small step at a time, and watch the path unveil itself. Don't be paralyzed by not having all the answers at once....because guess what...no one does.

The dawn of a new day brings a multitude of new possibilities. (Well, maybe they don't come at dawn....that is too early for my tastes.) Chances to begin anew. Chances to set a new goal or dream a new dream. You are never too young or too old for it. We are all given a finite number of days on Earth. Cancer makes you acutely aware of that. So go be happy. Get healthy. Live your dreams. Don't sit around and wait for good things to happen. Go make them happen. Use your gifts.

I have never been very evangelical. In fact, I am fairly private when it comes to the matter of spirituality. These things I know, though...I am drawn by both the quiet voice in my head and by the feeling in my soul. I am certain that this is the quiet, guiding voice of God. I believe we are used in different ways according to our gifts. We aren't all meant to shout from the rooftops. Some may share their special talents in a far more quiet and subtle way. We are all meant to go out and do good in the world. We are all designed to touch others with our special knacks and talents. Every time you share your gifts, a little more good is revealed from inside of you. A spark is released, and that positive energy can create a ripple effect capable of changing the world.

So what are you waiting for?

Go on.....vamoose....get out there...and LIVE.

Eleven

Life Keeps Moving

October 2014 - Epilogue

Well, it is almost my two year Cancerversary, praise the Lord! My big six month checkup with my oncologist is just around the corner. Of course, it comes with a bit of scanxiety. I feel in my heart that I am healthy, but cancer can be sneaky and stealth like a spider…and I hate spiders! I saw my breast surgeons last week. On the cancer front, no new lumps or bumps which is very positive news. However, my foobs need some maintenance. Despite massage, exercise, and stretching, I have some serious contracture problems that will require a new surgery to fix. Recall that my implants are encased in between the muscles in my chest wall. There is a band of muscle tissue across each implant that has formed a permanent hard capsule causing deformity and pain. The fix will involve opening my old scars, performing a capsulotomy on the affected muscle tissue, and removing my current implants. I will get a new set of foobs which will be a different kind of implant. Hopefully this will fix the problems! Aye yai yai….I will have DRAINS again. Yikes!

See- I told you reconstruction is not a boob job. This will be the seventh time in 24 months that my chest will be cut.

What else have I been up to this year? I have begun seeing Pilates clients in my small home studio…and I love it! Let's see… what else? I had my remaining girl parts removed in February. I am now void of two boobs, two ovaries, one uterus, and one cervix. No ovaries also means that I am extremely lacking in estrogen. Man am I thankful for fashion and lipstick to keep me feeling girly!

Also, after eighteen months out of the recommended five years, I have developed an intolerance to my anti-cancer meds. I was taking an aromatase inhibitor to keep my body from converting other substances into estrogen. The medicine caused joint pain, insomnia, hot flashes, and more. Though not fun, I was able to choke it down every day because I knew that it was proven to help ward off more cancer. However, when the side effects turned into an allergic reaction, I had to nix it (per doctor's orders). I was experiencing dizziness, itching and facial swelling. My oncologist switched me to another medication in the same class; aaaaaaand the same thing happened. I am sure we will discuss all of this during my upcoming appointment, but for now, I am focusing on healthy lifestyle choices.

The cancer road goes on forever and the party never ends!

Other than that, keeping up with my precious family and writing this book has kept me very busy. David is still in and out of the country. Maggie has begun high school, and she is growing into a fantastic artist. Sarah Jayne is in seventh grade; playing volleyball and loving science like her mama. Genevieve is taking pre-school by storm. I got some ink…a big lion head with a pink lotus flower and pink ribbon in the mane. "Roar" inspired: "I got the eye of the tiger, a fighter, dancing through the fire, 'Cause I am a champion and you're gonna hear me roar. Louder, louder than a lion….." Katy Perry.

Oh wait! I almost forgot about First Descents! Ohmylordwhatafantasticexperience. "What is First Descents?", you ask. It is a program that provides all-expenses paid adventure trips for young adult (under age 40) cancer fighters and survivors. We are talking week-long rock climbing, kayaking, and surfing trips.

Their motto is "Out Living It", and I cannot fully express what an empowering experience it was. My adventure was a rock climbing camp in Estes Park, Colorado. I went expecting to feel revived by the beauty of nature along with simply from taking a break from my everyday grind. Though those were both great, it was my experience with the people there that left me forever changed. The guides and volunteers were incredible. The campers were magnificent. The group was a motley crew with differing personalities, diagnoses, missing body parts, and prognoses….but

we all had a few things in common. One - cancer. And two - A
hell bent dedication to living life out loud despite our cancer.

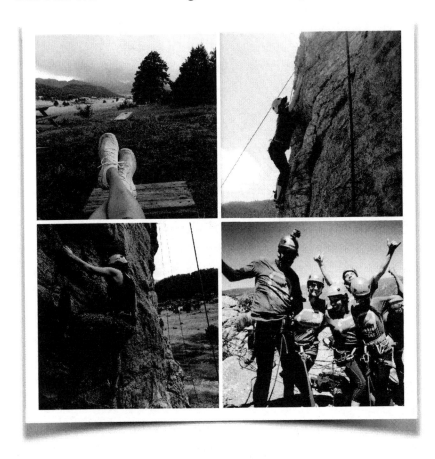

Boom! By the end of the week, I saw every single camper push
beyond their pre-conceived notions of their limitations. It was
such a worthy and amazing experience.

So, two years later, the dust is settling and a new normal is
emerging. I just went for my latest checkup (2 years from
diagnosis…), and I *finally* received a clear PET scan….no nodes lit
it up….hoooray! Though I am presently NED (No Evidence of
Disease), and so very grateful to say that, I am reminded that life is
neither the same nor as simple as it was before cancer. I find that

though I am scarred, I am definitely smarter. Smarter about love, life, and health.

As for this book, what began as a cathartic cancer memoir has grown into more. *Philosophically*, I really do believe that things happen for a reason...and that we can find meaning in our suffering. But *physiologically*, I wanted to know how I got cancer at age 36. No family history. No BRCA mutations. No acute risk factors. So, I began to research. As my research deepened, I became hungry to know not only why *I* got cancer, but why the incidence of many cancers is on the rise. In the second half of the book, I'll share with you what I found.

I have mentioned before that after a cancer diagnosis, friendships shift. Some friends disappear, other friendships strengthen, and a whole new circle of friends develops. This new circle is filled with other people who are waging their own war against cancer. Sadly, in the past year, the cancer circle has changed because some of those friends have lost their lives to this ugly, painful, expensive disease that does not discriminate. All of this fuels my desire for answers. I hope and pray that in our lifetime, we will witness the discovery of a cancer cure. Equally as important to me is that we learn how to PREVENT cancer from happening in the first place. My research makes me feel strongly that the chemical shit storm in which we live is wreaking havoc on the collective health of the human race and the planet in general. And not only in the context of cancer...but also in terms of autoimmune disorders, behavior disorders, reproductive issues, allergies, and more.

I urge you to read the second half of the book for a glimpse at how I have grown smarter about health. With time, I know that I will learn more and more. I am a forever-student. From the bottom of my heart, I thank you for taking the time to read about my little corner of the world. I hope that you discovered something of worth in all those chapters!

XOXO - *Natalie*
It is well. It is well with my soul.

Epilogue to the Epilogue
Because it is taking me much longer to finish this book than I anticipated!

December 11, 2014.....Dèjá vu. Two years to the very day of my bilateral mastectomy, I once again find myself at MD Anderson in the pre-op area awaiting surgery. It is time for my reconstruction re-do. I am in my hospital gown, which always makes me feel small and vulnerable. I can never quite get past the fact that I will soon be deprived of power, autonomy, and awareness; completely in the hands and at the mercy of others.

But then, the Chaplain comes to see me and together we pray. My soul is soothed, and I am ready. Surrender. Various doctors and nurses come and do their pre-op things. I am able to visit with my mom and Sarah Jayne....my caretakers for this surgery since David is in Afghanistan. We spend time talking about the anesthesia plan and the hope for no nausea. Before I know it, they are wheeling me down the hall. The drill is the same as it always is: people swirling around the operating room until I am knocked into a very deep sleep. Hours pass. My surgeon tells my mom that the surgery went well. He said that my tissue was like a sponge filled with water. I had tons of edema that had built up because of the capsulated scar tissue problem....both of which were addressed during surgery. He said that it was very obvious why I had been in quite a bit of pain. Glad to know it wasn't just in my head!

I wake dry-heaving. Dammit! I didn't escape my old enemy nausea this time. They pump me full of meds which greatly helps, but knocks me into a deep, deep sleep. It is all sort of hazy, but at some point I am discharged and my mom and Sarah Jayne wheel me to our room in the Rotary House. Now this is where it gets really funny. It is time for me to take a potty break, and my mom is supporting my hobble the restroom. I am only a step or two from the potty when she half-hollers, "You're gonna have to sit down!" while she simultaneously grabs the trash can and vomits! Dear Lord, she has food poisoning or a stomach virus. You can't make this stuff up! We both feel plain awful, but the situation is so ludicrous that it makes us laugh and laugh and laugh. We are curled up in our respective hotel beds...in pain and laughing like lunatics. The whole night is pretty miserable, but thankfully my sweet Sarah Jayne takes care of both of us. That child came into the world an old soul, and the past few years have revealed the reason why.

Breathe in. Breathe out.

Time once again to heal.

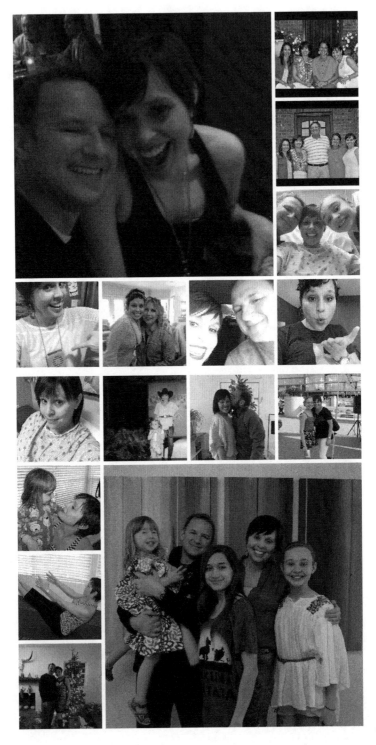

Part Two

The Get Healthy Manifesto

Twelve

Eyes Opened

Eyes Opened

Part One was all about my personal experience with cancer; the scarring that made way for the smarter. Part Two is all about the smarter. It is about all of the things I uncovered in my quest for answers. It is about being more aware and more in control of your own health.

I did not begin with any intention for this to be a two-part book, but it evolved into exactly that. I learned so many things that I want you to know as well. Having a health crisis as big as cancer hit me in my 30s made me take a long, hard look at my lifestyle. I realized that there were some lies I had been telling myself for years. Things like: "Thin equals healthy."..."I exercise, so I can eat whatever I want."... "Feeling exhausted is normal. I am a working mom." There were many other lies, too. Only these lies were the falsehoods lurking in plain sight camouflaged by the crafty marketing of the food, drug, and personal care product industries.

I found that there are so many sneaky ingredients in our environment, especially in our personal care products and in our food. We are bombarding ourselves daily with things that affect our health in a negative way. Think of it like this...your body is very complex and each part of it is designed to carry out very specific jobs. In the particular case of your immune system, you have many cells dedicated to attacking foreign substances to keep you healthy. So think of it as a war scenario with those protective cells equalling soldiers in combat. Their job is to protect against the bad guys. What if they were in the middle of a battle, and someone kept dropping bags of trash on them? That in itself is distracting, and when the trash piled high enough, they'd have to divert time and energy to to clearing the trash before they could even think about fighting their battle. The same is true in your body. If it is constantly being bombarded with garbage, it can't function in the way it is supposed to. Both chronic diseases and cancer can arise from of perfect storm genetics and of bodily insults from poor nutrition, to stress, to pollution. In order to give your body its best chance for good health, we definitely have to address toxic load and nutrition. That is exactly what Part Two is about. It will help you identify the toxins hiding in your daily routine so that you can identify them and replace them with healthier alternatives.

Part Two includes three chapters: Endocrine Disrupting Chemicals, Food, and Natural Health. Endocrine disrupting chemicals are particularly scary because they affect our hormones. Since hormones play a role almost every biochemical reaction in your body, things that alter them can have a huge impact on overall health. Then we have food - which is pretty important - because without it, we'd be dead. We will look at the good, the bad and the ugly as far as food is concerned. The last chapter is a short introduction to natural health. When it comes to health, as an American society, we have moved so far away from the natural approach as a first line of defense. We tend to assume that healthcare as it exists today is our only option. However, many other safe alternative and complementary approaches exist.

It is my hope that you will learn something new in each of the chapters that follow, and that you will use that information as a springboard for your own exploration of health.

Had I been totally in tune to all of the information in Part Two, Part One may have read much differently.

Hindsight…always twenty-twenty, right?

Thirteen

Endocrine Disrupting Chemicals

ENDOCRINE DISRUPTORS

If we are going to talk about things that disrupt the endocrine system, we must first talk a bit about the endocrine system itself. Your endocrine system is a network of glands in charge of sending hormones into the circulatory system. I find that when I mention the word 'hormone', most people immediately think of estrogen and testosterone, as if they are THE only hormones. Not so! Hormones extend well beyond sex-specific hormones, and they are muy importante! Think of hormones as bossy. Since they serve as messengers and communicators telling your body when to do what, how much to do it, and how often to do it, they control pretty much everything. Your endocrine system uses biofeedback to control the release of hormones. The major players in the endocrine system include the pineal gland, pituitary gland, pancreas, ovaries, testes, thyroid gland, parathyroid gland, hypothalamus, gastrointestinal tract, and adrenal glands. They monitor the release of hormones which allow cells, tissues, and organs to talk to one another. Hormones then regulate digestion, metabolism, respiration, tissue function, sensory perception, sleep, excretion, lactation, stress, growth, development, movement, reproduction, and mood.....in other words, hormones affect close to every action in your body. If they are out of balance, a host of unfortunate things from the unsatisfactory to the down right miserable can result. Ergo, things that interfere with the endocrine system play a crucial role in our health.

Enter endocrine disruptors, aka EDCs (Endocrine Disrupting Chemicals). The NIH (National Institutes of Health) describes endocrine disruptors as "substances that may interfere with the body's endocrine system and produce adverse developmental, reproductive, neurological, and immune effects in both humans and wildlife". (1) We live in a world in which man-made chemicals have become a part of everyday life. More industrialization has brought more EDCs. Currently, around

80,000 chemicals exist on the market in the United States, many of which are used by millions of Americans in their daily lives. The vast majority of these chemicals are either understudied or not studied at all and are largely unregulated. That isn't a typo....EIGHTY THOUSAND CHEMICALS.....MANY OF WHICH ARE NOT EVEN STUDIED. (2) A large number of these 80,000 chemicals did not exist before World War I. Now they are present everywhere....in our food....shampoo...body lotion...clothing....furniture....and more. The typical American is exposed to around 125 different chemicals each day through their *personal care products alone.* (3) This number DOES NOT include chemicals from *other* environmental exposures, chemicals in the workplace, chemicals in food, chemicals in modern lifestyle products, or chemicals from medical sources.

Synthetic chemicals are so ubiquitous in our environment, even our *babies are born pre-polluted.* Tiny, sweet, have-never-even-drawn-a-breath babies are born with several HUNDRED chemicals in their cord blood. Of the 287 chemicals detected in umbilical cord blood, 180 are known to cause cancer in humans or animals, 217 are toxic to the brain and nervous system, and 208 cause birth defects or abnormal development in animal tests. Exposure during fetal development can lead to problems later in life: learning disabilities, ADHD, cancer, and more. It is no wonder that we are seeing increases in all of these. The Environmental Working Group explains it well by saying, "Chemical exposures in the womb or during infancy can be dramatically *more* harmful than exposures later in life. Substantial scientific evidence demonstrates that children face amplified risks from their body burden of pollution; the findings are particularly strong for many of the chemicals found in this study, including mercury, PCBs and dioxins. Children's vulnerability derives from both rapid development and incomplete defense systems:

- A developing child's chemical exposures are greater pound-for-pound than those of adults.

- An immature, porous blood-brain barrier allows greater chemical exposures to the developing brain.
- Children have lower levels of some chemical-binding proteins, allowing more of a chemical to reach "target organs."
- A baby's organs and systems are rapidly developing, and thus are often more vulnerable to   damage from chemical exposure.
- Systems that detoxify and excrete industrial chemicals are not fully developed.
- The longer future life span of a child compared to an adult allows more time for adverse effects to arise." (4)

How frightening is that? We are being bombarded with so many EDCs daily, that even our babies are not protected in the womb. ~~Americans~~ People of the Planet, we MUST change our ways. We can't get to it fast enough.

Numerous sources of endocrine disrupting chemicals include: pharmaceuticals, dioxin and dioxin-like compounds, polychlorinated biphenyls, DDT and other pesticides, plasticizers (such as but not limited to BPA), and in everyday products– including plastic bottles, metal food cans, detergents, flame retardants, food, toys, baby toys, cosmetics, and pesticides. Endocrine disruptors may have negative effects at any point in the lifespan, but seem to pose the greatest risk during pregnancy, early post-natal development, and puberty. (5)

A 2012 large-scale review collaboration by the United Nations Environment Programme (UNEP) and the World Health Organization (WHO) sought to address the concerns about the adverse effects of EDCs. Understand that when I say large-scale, I mean it. This wasn't just one small study. It involved the work of 21 scientists from around the globe, and it references 18 MAJOR studies. Review of the studies showed that there is both emerging and mounting evidence for adverse reproductive outcomes (infertility, cancers, malformations); disrupted thyroid and brain functions; and unfavorable effects on obesity, metabolism, insulin and glucose homeostasis. (6)

Since more than 50 different hormones and hormone-related molecules in humans integrate and control normal body functions throughout the lifespan, you can see how anything which disrupts them can cause a major fiasco. Cancer is not the only resulting disaster. We are talking everything from......ahem, listen up men....reductions in male fertility and declines in the numbers of males born (and not just for human males...but also in the animal kingdom in general) to abnormalities in male reproductive organs. Ladies: tune in...endocrine disrupters are linked to fertility problems, early puberty, and early menopause. As for issues affecting both the guys and the gals: increases in certain cancers, increases in immune and autoimmune diseases, and some neurodegenerative diseases are linked to endocrine disruptors. (7) The dysfunction of the immune system caused by EDCs may lead immunodeficiency against infection or hyper-reactivity of immune responses (in other words: autoimmune diseases and allergies). (8)

  As you are reading this, you may be trying to convince yourself that none of this applies to you since you only get a little of this and a little of that. If so, let me try to shift your perspective by highlighting two things that really stand out to me. First- little things can have big effects. Think about this....there is one tiny pill I take daily. It is designed to prevent a cancer relapse. It is itty bitty....smaller than a chocolate chip, but powerful. I feel the effects of it every day through waves of hot flashes, insomnia, and serious pain in my joints. Little pill; low dose; grande effects. So lesson number one is: when dealing with hormones, a little bit can have far reaching effects. The dose does not make the poison. As for lesson two, let's talk cocktails. Not Mai Tais and Mojitos, but EDCs. There are little bits of those suckers everywhere - in the pesticides on your food, in the flame retardants clothing or furniture, in the additives and preservatives in your shampoo, lotion, shave gel, and makeup, in your food packaging, in your sunscreen, and more. When you look at a study of a small amount of a particular EDC, the results may lead one to believe that they are relatively safe. However, when you look at studies which combine little bits of many different EDCs, the results are disastrous. (6) Alcohol....an antihistamine...a valium...a pain killer...a small amount of each on its own has a certain effect, but combine them....and you are in a world of trouble. The same holds true for EDCs....a little here...plus a smidgen there...and another dash or two throughout the day....day in....day out...week after week....month after month....year after year....hope you get the picture.

Let's take a look at your exposures....before breakfast:

The alarm sounds, you may snooze a few more minutes, then you roll out of bed...out of your sheets that have enveloped you all night in detergent, fabric softener, and bleach. (A,B,C,D,E,F,G) You walk bleary eyed to the bathroom, turn on the shower, and douse your body with soap/body wash (C,D,E,F,G,H,I), shampoo (A,D,H,I), conditioner (A,D,I), facial cleanser (C,D,H,I), and shave creme (C,D,H,I). Now it is time for moisturizer (A,C,D,E,F,G,H), skin rash/acne medication (A,C,D,E,F,G,H), cologne/perfume (A,D,G,H,I), antiperspirant/deodorant (A,D,E,F,G,H), hairspray (D,G), toothpaste (C,D,E,F,I), and mouthwash (D,E,F,H,I). Time for more as you doll up with foundation, blush, eyeshadow, lipstick, and mascara (A,C,D,G,H,I). Throw on your dry-cleaned clothes (A,G) and hit the kitchen for a soda (D,F,H,I) or some coffee with artificial sweetener (I) and GMO milk/creamer (F). Doh! There is a rumble in your tummy, so you must hit the bathroom after which you fumigate it with air freshener (A,D,G,H).

Wondering why you may feel bad? Have chronic digestive or skin issues? Feel fatigued? Have a hard time concentrating? Check out what you what you just loaded your body with...and you haven't even had breakfast yet!

A. Alcohols–Acid & Alkali: rashes, muscle weakness, headaches, dizziness, nerve damage, vision problems, sleeping problems, stomach cramps, disorientation, depression, coughing, respiratory problems, anemia, organ damage, fatigue, heart damage, cancer, death.

B. Chlorines: headaches, mental function difficulties, pulmonary edemas and heart disease, anemia, diabetes, gastrointestinal and urinary tract cancer, organ and gland cancer, severe eye problems, immune system breakdown, child development problems and more.

C. Detergents/Emulsifiers: strip skin of protective oils, skin irritation, scalp eruptions, interference with nutrient absorption, hair loss, allergic reaction, cataract formation, organ damage, reproductive damage, blindness, cancer.

D. Synthetic Fragrance & Dyes: allergic reactions, skin rashes, stomach upsets, muscular aches and pains, violent coughing and sneezing, irritability, vertigo, hyperactivity, convulsions, emotional and behavioral problems, Leukemia, Hodgkin's, emotional problems, ADD, multiple tumors, reproductive damage, headaches, dizziness, organ damage, depression, cancer.

E. Heavy Metals: Abdominal cramps, nausea, joint and bone pain, muscle weakness, mouth sores, muscle, joint, and bone pain; cancer, motor difficulties, reduced intelligence, brain disorders, short attention span, hyperactivity, short attention span, emotional disorders, immune disorders, genetic damage, aging.

F. Pesticides & Fungicides: Flu-like symptoms (fatigue, muscle and joint pain),stomach cramps, nervous system disorders, insomnia, memory loss, swelling of body parts, dizziness, genetic mutations, birth defects, gland tumors, organ damage, cancers, death.

G. Petrochemicals: inhibit skin functions, pimples, rashes, splitting nails, sensitivity to sun, headaches, premature aging, allergic reactions, depression, fatigue, intestinal gas, asthma, respiratory failure, immune system disorders.

H. Preservatives (synthetic): headaches, shin rashes, eye damage, asthma, respiratory problems, tumors, cancer, digestive problems, mental confusion, organ damage, muscle weakness & cramps, loss of motor control, joint pain, reproductive damage, etc.

I. Artificial flavors, colors, preservatives: allergies, asthma, hay fever, hyperactivity, rashes, nausea, vomiting

(Inspired by: The Politics of Poison by Nina G. Silver, Ph.D., 2000, government agencies, and medical institutions, and product manufacturers)

And that is just the morning routine. Now, consider all the other ways you are exposed throughout the day. It is estimated that today we are exposed to more chemicals in one month than our grandparents were throughout their lifetime. There is no time like RIGHT THIS MINUTE to begin making the switch to a more natural way of life.

Exactly *how* do endocrine disruptors work? They can act as **mimickers** of naturally occurring hormones. This means they act like estrogens, androgens, and thyroid hormones potentially producing overstimulation. They can be **binders,** meaning they spot a receptor on a cell and beat the real hormone to it. As such, the actual hormone cannot bind to the cell and the message it needed to give the cell gets lost. When this happens, the body cannot respond properly or activate cycles that need to occur. Since binding EDCs block or antagonize real hormones, they are also known as anti-estrogens and anti-androgens. Finally, EDCs can also **disrupt the production** of hormones. EDCs can change the way real hormones are metabolized in the liver leading to a shortage of certain hormones. (*1*)

So, we have established that EDCs are really bad; really really bad. One hundred percent bad news. Want to know what takes the whole situation next-level? There are no current U.S. laws which address endocrine disrupting chemicals. None. After reading this, I hope they are on your radar and that you do all that is in your power to avoid the bulk of them. Need a CliffNote version to help you identify some of the most commonly found EDCs? Here you go:

PCBs and Dioxins

THE LOWDOWN: Mainly by-products of industrial processes like smelting, chlorine bleaching of paper pulp, and the manufacture of herbicides and pesticides, though some occurs naturally through volcanic eruptions and forrest fires. 90% of human exposure is from the food supply, mainly from meat, dairy, fish and shellfish. (These chemicals bioaccumulate…meaning that they are stored in fatty tissues and that their concentration increases as you move up the food chain.)

REDUCE EXPOSURE by trimming fat on meat and choosing lower fat dairy items. Eat an abundance of organic fruits and veggies. (*9*)

Flame Retardants
(Polybrominated flame retardants, PDBEs)

THE LOWDOWN: Electronics, plastics, textiles, car interiors and many other products contain chemical fire suppressors. You may be thinking, well then, it is nearly impossible to limit my exposure to flame retardants then. Not true. In North America, meat, poultry, dairy and fish are known to be contaminated with flame retardants. The food comes into contact with them during processing and through packaging materials. High-fat poultry and red meat were associated with higher blood serum levels of flame retardants. Vegetarians had around 25% lower serum levels. (*10*)

Let's not forget BVO (brominated vegetable oil) is present in many citrus flavored soft drinks and in sports drinks like Gatorade and Powerade (though the makers of Gatorade have pledged to remove it). BVO was approved by the FDA in the 1970s and is still on the GRAS (Generally Recognized as Safe) list despite numerous studies since then outlined the risks. "BVO exposure has caused reproductive damage; neurological damage; severe behavioral problems; and permanent organ damage to the heart, kidneys, and testicles" in animal studies. It is outlawed as a food additive in over 100 countries, and Europe, Japan, India and others are working to ban its use as a plasticizer all together. (*11*) PDBEs accumulate in the liver, kidneys, and thyroid gland, and are known endocrine disruptors.

REDUCING EXPOSURE to PDBEs in electronics, textiles, cars, and household furniture may be challenging. When buying new furniture, opt for those without retardants. Reducing food exposure can be done by eating more plants than animals or being vegetarian....and by all means.....avoid those toxic soft and sports drinks containing BVO. Do you really want to drink flame retardants? Opt for water...water with a splash of fruit.....organic coffee or tea. Last but not least, no need for flame retardants in clothing. When choosing pajamas, opt for sustainable fabrics. (For children, choose snug-fitting cotton jammies.)

Pesticides

THE LOWDOWN: The very design of pesticides allows them to disrupt biological processes. After all, that is how they kill plants and pests. So it stands to reason that they may be harmful to humans, too. Some kill by disrupting cellular processes thereby resulting in death; others act on the hormone system of plants and insects. Adverse effects on humans can happen at low doses. The effects can alter the signaling systems that control both function and development. Parental exposure can even effect subsequent generations (epigenetics). Scary. (*12*) "Pesticides, including their presumed inert ingredients, are among a growing list of chemicals demonstrated to interfere with sexual development, reproduction, and fertility when exposure occurs during vulnerable life stages." (*13*) This is another incidence where exposure at low doses can have effects that may not be immediately noticeable, rather they manifest over a period of time.

The best way to REDUCE EXPOSURE is by buying non-GMO and organic foods. We'll dig much deeper into this topic in the food chapter.

Perfluorinated chemicals (PFCs)

THE LOWDOWN: PFCs are a large group of manufactured compounds that are widely used to make everyday products more resistant to stains, grease, and water. You can find them in grease-resistant food packaging and paper products, such as microwave popcorn bags and pizza boxes. They were used until 2002 in 3M's Scotchgard® used on carpet, furniture, and clothing. PFCs are used to make DuPont's Teflon™'s famous non-stick cookware. They can even be found in personal care products like shampoo, dental floss, make-up and denture cleaners (look for ingredients with words containing "fluoro" or "perfluoro"). Studies have linked PFCs to cancer, low birth weight, reproductive problems, behavioral issues including ADHD, and reduced vaccine immune protection in children. (*14,15*) Here is another alarming fact about PFCs: their half-life in the human body ranges from around 4 years to around 8 years. That means that once there is uptake into your body, it takes a minimum of four years for HALF of that amount to decay and be excreted. Then it takes another 4 years for HALF of that remaining amount to break down and leave your body....and so on.

You can REDUCE EXPOSURE and stop PFCs from building up in your body by avoiding purchasing or at least limiting use of products containing PFC ingredients. Stay away from greasy processed foods and fast foods since their packaging often contains grease-repellant PFC coatings. Limit your purchases of "stain resistant" products. Check your personal care products and cosmetics. Avoid Teflon™ or non-stick cookware. If you cannot chunk it all at once, over time replace it piece by piece. Start by getting rid of the pieces showing scratches or signs of deterioration.

Phthalates

THE LOWDOWN: We are surrounded by phthalates. They are often referred to as plasticizers and they are added to products to make them flexible. You can find them in PVC products such as vinyl flooring, vinyl shower curtains, and children's toys. They are in tons of personal care products such as shampoos, body washes, perfumes, nail polishes, and lotions. They are found in many medical devices like IV bags and tubing. Automobile interiors contain them, and they are present in our air, water, and soil due to industrial pollution form leaching and from consumer products. (16) Studies have shown that we definitely absorb phthalates from our personal care products. (17) Please think twice before you slather yourself with phthalate-containing shampoos, conditioners, lotions, makeup, and other personal care products. What you put ON your body DOES matter, because it is absorbed. Higher phthalate exposure and absorption is also associated with fast food consumption. Again, it matters what you put IN your body. (18)

Yikes. It feels like there is no escaping phthalates. Here is the good news: they don't build up in your body. However, because our exposure is ubiquitous, a steady stream of them is present in our bodies. So if you can reduce your exposure, you can also reduce the amount that is always circulating in your body. Hooray for good news!

REDUCE EXPOSURE by avoiding PVC as much as you can and purchasing products from companies that have eliminated phthalates. If you can, avoid vinyl building products in your home (shower curtains, windows, doors, and flooring). You can avoid PVC packaging by looking for and avoiding the #3 recycling symbol. If it has the #3 symbol, then it contains PVC. Choose cotton shower curtains with a polyester or nylon liner instead of vinyl shower curtains. Many toys contain PVC. Companies that have pledged to stop using PVC include Early Start, Little Tikes, Lego, Prime Time Playthings, Sassy, and Tiny Love. Store food in glass containers when possible. And for the love of your health, DO NOT warm food in plastic. If you are using plastic wrap and bags, buy those made from polyethylene. Remember to avoid those products with the recycling symbol #3. (*16*)

BPA (Bisphenol A)
THE LOWDOWN: Found in polycarbonate plastics and epoxy resins. (Plastic bottles and containers, lining of canned vegetables and fruits.) Also, be aware that BPA has an evil twin: BPS. Bisphenol S is just as harmful. It has been found to both mimic estrogen and to increase the aggressiveness of breast cancer.

REDUCE EXPOSURE: Look for BPA free packaged items. Better yet, avoid plastics whenever possible. Do not warm food in plastic containers. (*1*)

UV Filters

THE LOWDOWN: Sunscreens. Though they are effective in preventing sunburns, their protective effects against melanoma skin cancer is less conclusive. Use of sunscreen worldwide is increasing, yet so is incidence of malignant melanoma. UV-filters are rapidly absorbed in the skin, and there is an increasing body of evidence pointing to their endocrine-disrupting actions.

REDUCE EXPOSURE by using sunscreen FREE of : oxybenzone, benzophenone-3 (BP-3), 3-benzylidene camphor (3-BC), 3-(4-methyl-benzylidene) camphor (4-MBC), 2-ethylhexyl 4-methoxy cinnamate (OMC), Homosalate (HMS), 2-ethylhexyl 4-dimethylaminobenzoate (OD-PABA) and 4-aminobenzoic acid (PABA). *(19)* Also, the sunscreen should be free of parabens and fragrance.

Triclosan

THE LOWDOWN: You can find this little gem in things like antibacterial soap, hand sanitizers, dish detergents, and even toothpaste. You can also find it in the bodies of over 75% of Americans over the age of 6....you can find it in human blood and even breastmilk. It is absorbed through the skin. This little beast has been proven to weaken both skeletal and cardiac muscle. *(19)* It was on the FDA's radar for over 35 years before a lawsuit by the National Resources Defense Council forced them to issue a final rule. Now, all hand soaps must be triclosan free by 2016. For me, this speaks VOLUMES. The FDA thought it was bad in 1978, YET it took 35 years AND a lawsuit for them to deem it unsafe for consumer use. If that doesn't tell you that you should be sticking to things that are as natural as possible, I don't know what would. It also speaks volumes about just how long it takes to see change in the personal care and cosmetic industry.

REDUCE EXPOSURE by avoiding all products containing triclosan.

Parabens

THE LOWDOWN: Parabens are used to prevent the growth of yeasts, molds, and bacteria in cosmetics products. Parabens appear in some deodorants and antiperspirants, in addition to personal care products that contain significant amounts of water, such as shampoos, conditioners, lotions, and facial and shower cleansers and scrubs. They're also widely used as preservatives in food and pharmaceutical products. Parabens are estrogen mimickers, and they are found in nearly all urine samples from U.S. adults of a variety of ethnic, socioeconomic and geographic backgrounds. (20)

A 2004 UK study detected traces of five different parabens in the breast tumors of 19 out of 20 women studied (21). This small study does not prove a causal relationship between parabens and breast cancer, but it *is* important because it detected the presence of intact parabens—unaltered by the body's metabolism. This is an indication of the chemical's ability to penetrate skin and remain in breast tissue. Since the parabens were completely intact, also shows that the human body is not able to break them down. A more recent study found higher levels of one paraben, n-propylparaben, in the axilla quadrant of the breast (the area nearest the underarm). This is the region in which the highest proportion of breast tumors are found. (22) Ongoing studies are looking at parabens as causative agents for breast cancer. Recent work has shown that **both parabens and BPA interfere with the effectiveness of anti-cancer drugs used in the treatment of breast cancer.** (23) Not only are parabens linked to cancer, but they are also related to reproductive toxicity, immunotoxicity, neurotoxicity and skin irritation (24, 25, 26, 27). Since parabens are used to kill bacteria in water-based solutions, they inherently have some toxicity to cells (28).

142

REDUCE EXPOSURE by being a label reader! Since most of us use a ton of personal care products, all of that label reading can seem daunting. There are many do-it-yourself options for personal care products. For the products I purchase, I buy from a small number of companies who make products free of parabens, phthalates, synthetic fragrances, and other petrochemicals.

BHA & BHT (Butylated Hydroxyanisole)

THE LOWDOWN: Based on animal studies, BHA and BHT have been classified as 'reasonable human carcinogens' since 1991, yet they are still present in a big way in our food supply as well as some makeup & personal care products. They are approved and allowed by the FDA in certain low concentrations per product. Remember - though the concentration per product may be low, it is the cumulative exposure from many different sources that is scary. A dash here and a smidgen there adds up! BHA and BHT are found in many processed, packaged foods and fried foods They are used as preservatives and anti-oxidants in pharmaceutical preparations and cosmetics containing fats and oils (especially eyeshadows and lipsticks). Use of BHA in the food industry in the United States tripled between 1960 and 1978. Since our consumption of pre-packaged and processed foods has sky-rocketed since then, I shudder to think about what those numbers may look like now. (29)

REDUCE EXPOSURE by …. once again …. being a label reader. You can greatly reduce your exposure by avoiding processed and pre-packed foods as much as possible. Additionally, avoid BHA and BHT in your personal care products.

Is your head spinning yet? I know, I know…it is a lot to digest. Did you have any idea you were exposing yourself to so many endocrine disrupting chemicals? Until I started doing my

143

research, I also had no idea how deep the rabbit hole went. I assumed that for the most part, consumer products were safe simply because they lined the shelves of my local Target, Walgreens, or beauty station at the mall.

Understandably, there is growing concern about the toxic effects of over-exposure to chemicals that appear in our environment. In this chapter, we have talked specifically about EDCs, but the toxic load in general has also been linked to everything from skin sensitivities, to allergies, to cancer. Only a few hundred of the 80,000 chemicals in use in the United States have been tested for safety. Much like the monitoring of the safety of food additives and GMOs (more about that in the following chapter), the approach to regulating environmental contaminants is more *reactionary* than *precautionary*. Instead of requiring the industry to prove the safety of chemicals, preservatives, fragrances, and additives; it is the general public who bears the burden of proving that a given environmental exposure is harmful. It is no wonder that the incidence of some cancers, including some most common among children, is increasing for unexplained reasons. (2)

So, I urge you:

DO NOT WAIT FOR THE BURDEN TO BE PROVEN.

Be proactive. Make changes. Choose health now.

You can also check out my blog at
www.YourHouseOfHealing.com
for new health articles and for links to
suggested healthier products.

Fourteen

Food

Food

Food. Could it play a larger or more important role in our lives? I mean without it…we'd be dead. Not only is it life sustaining, but food is deeply cultural as well…present in our family, holiday, celebration, and grieving traditions. In this chapter, we'll talk about the good, the bad, and the downright ugly when it comes to food. The great thing is that food has the ability to *nourish* us. The very definition of ***nourish*** is to provide the body with food and other substances necessary for **growth, health, and good condition.** Let that sink in for a minute. Food is supposed to sustain you. It can play a HUGE role in preventing disease and in maintaining & restoring health. Eons ago, Hippocrates knew how important food was when he said "Let thy food be thy medicine and medicine be thy food". Why is it that the emphasis on that has been so lost in recent years? Boxed, pre-packaged, and full of artificial flavors, colors, & preservatives; the typical "Western Diet" has morphed into something that is a far cry from "food". So much of what the general population eats today shouldn't even qualify as food. Food can nourish us, or it can serve as a very potent and and very slow poison…..and that is no exaggeration. Again, let that sink in. When you eat junk, (and we'll talk about what constitutes junk in a bit) you are pouring in **calories** and **chemicals.** This fills you up with things void of the vitamins, minerals, amino acids, and other necessary building blocks for health.

As for the food safety and dietary recommendations in this country, the approach is more reactive than proactive - just like it is with chemicals in our personal care products and the environment. We are being duped by the big wigs every single day, and frankly I am sick of it. High-dollar advertising campaigns keep food lies hidden in plain sight. I find it disturbing that it takes public outcry for any changes to be made. There is an easy way to speak loudly, though. As with anything, follow the money trail, and you will see who is in control of our food. That money trail is a two-way street.

If you want to send a message way up the totem pole, then speak when you spend. Stop buying their lies and their faux-food, and eventually they will get the picture. Okay - - - you may be picking up on the fact that this is a VERY hot topic for me. You are right. We have the ability to be in control of so much when it comes to our health. I understand that making lifestyle and diet changes can seem daunting and overwhelming. I get it, I really do. However, if you are interested in taking charge of your own health and the health of your family, then it is absolutely imperative. It is absolutely worth it as well. Some choose to make fast and dramatic changes. They pull out the garbage can, dump all the crap and start fresh. Others choose to make small changes over time, exchanging one bad habit for a good one until their whole routine has been overhauled. You have to choose what is right for you. Either way, you are making positive changes and moving in the right direction. Go ahead and give yourself a big pat on the back! Let's talk about the bad stuff first so we can finish on a good note.

THE BAD AND UGLY

"The modern diet is the main reason why people all over the world are **fatter** and **sicker** than ever before. Everywhere modern processed foods go, chronic diseases like obesity, Type II diabetes, and heart disease soon follow."

-Author Kris Gunnars

("I couldn't agree more!"
-Natalie Holland)

SUGAR CONSUMPTION

Sugar consumption for the average American increased by around 20% between 1970 and 2005. (1) Today, the majority of this increase is in the form processed sugar and corn syrup. (Much of which is from GMO crops. More later on GMO crops.) That's a lot of empty *and* inflammatory calories, y'all. A huge source of all this added sugar is from soda, fruit juices, and other sweetened drinks. Multiple studies have shown that such sweet beverages dramatically increase your risk of metabolic syndrome (aka pre-diabetes), Type II diabetes, heart disease, and mortality. (2) Now 'merica, don't take that as an excuse to use artificial sweeteners, because they are also detrimental to your health. Studies show that they lead to even greater weight gain! When it comes to beverages, you cannot beat good ole water. Add a few drops of citrus essential oils of your choice for flavor and to stimulate gentle detoxification. Or toss in a few fruit slices. If you must sweeten your beverages, choose a small amount of organic local honey or some agave syrup. If you are baking, these two are also good in place of refined sugar. Pure organic stevia (with no additives) is a good choice as well. (Liquid is better as powdered versions are heavily processed.)

American dietary guidelines recommend no more than 8 teaspoons per day of added sugar in the diet. Aaaaaand we presently consume, on average, around 30 teaspoons of added sugar per day. Yikes! For the sake of our overall health, we need to scale back. (1) So put down that sticky bun and grab a piece of fruit or a handful of nuts.

ISOCALORIC vs ISOMETABOLIC
PROCESSED OILS AND SUGARS

First notice that the heading for this section includes our old foe "processed". Seeing a trend here? So, I am pretty sure you know what processed means, but what about isocaloric and isometabolic. Iso means "same", so basically what this means is that though two food sources may have the *same* number of *calories*, the *metabolic effect* of the two foods is entirely *different*. All of this is well explained by Dr. Robert Lustig, MD, University of California, San Francisco, School of Medicine specialist on pediatric hormone disruptors and leading expert in childhood obesity. Take high-fructose corn syrup (HFCS) for example. It is a highly processed mixture of both glucose and fructose. HFCS is primarily metabolized by the liver while glucose *in its natural form* is metabolized by every cell in the body. When fructose hits the liver in a fast dose, as with processed HFCS....especially when in liquid form as in processed juices and sodas, the liver converts much of it directly to fat. The case is different with glucose and fructose obtained from pure fruit sources, as the fiber in them helps the body metabolize them at a much slower rate. *(3)* All of this gives me flashbacks to my nutritional biochemistry classes. Your body is such an amazing and extremely complex miracle of a machine. Something becomes of every morsel you put into your mouth. *Real* food can be broken down and used by the body for nourishment. However, in the case of processed food, it cannot always be broken down and assimilated by the body. Some by-products are excreted while others that cannot be processed hang around and cause all sorts of damage. Though your body's design is incredibly intricate, when you look at the evidence, one thing is pretty simple: it isn't designed to handle the load of processed chemical crap we tend to feed it.

    Processed sugar is not the only thing about which to worry. Processed oils play a huge detrimental role in our diets as well. You can blame this public-health-experiment-gone-wrong on the Low Fat Lie. (See the next section) First of all, your body benefits from healthy fats. You need them for proper brain function (especially developing infants and toddlers), and they help you absorb fat soluble vitamins A, D, E, and K. However; and most unfortunately, healthy saturated fats have long been portrayed as villainous while low-fat alternatives such as corn oil, canola oil, and margarine have been portrayed as healthy. Well. *That is just absolutely wrong.* After years and years the FDA is finally admitting it. The Centers for Disease Control estimates that 7000 deaths and 20,000 heart attacks per year could be prevented by removing the majority of trans fats from the food supply….and the FDA is on board. (4)

So what makes those low-fat oils so bad? Several things. Let's start with the fact that they are hydrogenated. Hydrogenated oils are made by adding a hydrogen to a polyunsaturated oil. This process makes the oil cheaper and less perishable. Here we go again with the money trail…cheaper products equal more profits for the big dogs. So why is this bad for your body? A very quick (I promise!) chemistry lesson will explain. Here goes: structurally, an unsaturated oil has a zigzag like structure. Your body is full of fats like this….namely your cell membranes….and that structure helps to provide fluidity. BUT, when you take one of those unsaturated oils and hydrogenate it…though it still has a zigzag like structure, it is the *mirror image opposite* of that of an unsaturated oil….and this is where the name "trans" fat comes from. So now you have something your body has a hard time grabbing, thereby making it impossible for it to incorporate hydrogenated trans fats into cell structures. Those trans fats become like puzzle pieces that won't fit. Not only is your body unable to properly use such fats, but it also has a hard time excreting them. This means they build up in your body and just circulate in your blood causing all sorts of mischief like heart disease and cancer. (5) Not only do trans-fats clog up arteries and more, they can also transform the ratio of omega 6 to omega 3 fatty acids to an unhealthy state. Your body needs both of these fats, and the optimal ratio is 1:1. The ratio in the typical Western diet is around 15:1. This imbalance promotes "the pathogenesis of many diseases, including cardiovascular disease, cancer, and inflammatory and autoimmune diseases". (6) Cooking oils are not the only culprits of the omega6/omega3 imbalance. Grain fed animals have added to the fatty-acid flip flop in beef, chicken, and dairy products. "When humans were hunter-gatherers, diets consisted mostly of wild plants, fruits, leafy green vegetables, fish, and meat from *grazing animals*. The eventual switch in domestic animal feed from grass and hay to omega-6–rich grains changed the fatty acid composition of the animals' meat and dairy products accordingly." (7) Bringing the omega 3 and omega 6 fatty acid ratio into balance not only reduces the risks for cardiovascular disease, cancer, inflammatory and immune diseases, but it also helps trim the fat from our bodies. (8) This is one of the reasons that it is important to choose grass-fed meat & dairy products and healthy cooking oils.

LOW-FAT LIES

Raise your hand if you have long believed that a healthy diet is a low-fat diet. Did most of you shoot up your arm? I did. I grew up thinking that low fat = healthy because that is what marketing told my mama (and me as I grew into adulthood) to believe. I remember filling the grocery cart with Snackwell's low-fat cookies, newtons, and more. Full of sugar, but low in fat! These "Snackwell's" snacks didn't evolve in grandma's kitchen with good old fashioned ingredients. Instead they were created in a lab by food scientist Sam Porcello. How about all of those Lean Cuisines and Healthy Choice low calorie and low fat microwavable dinners? Have you looked at the ingredient list? If you have, you'll know that the list is long (red flag) and full of words that sound nothing like food. I die a little on the inside when I think about the decade I spent teaching high school and just how many times I nuked 'healthy' meals in PLASTIC containers in the microwave. Dear Lord.

There are many other cleverly marketed products I can recall, but I cannot move on before mentioning "Olean" and "Wow" chips. If these conjure a memory for you, it is probably accompanied by a churn in your stomach. These doozies contained Olestra, which was discovered by Proctor and Gamble. As an additive, Olestra prevents your body from absorbing fat.....but that comes with a price. Mal-absorption of fat-soluble vitamins A, D, E, and K. Abdominal cramping. Loose stools. Anal leakage.

Anybody singing… *"When you're sliding into first and you feel a sudden burst…"* Just keep humming along…

The FDA wouldn't approve Olestra as a DRUG, but they did approve it as a FOOD ADDITIVE. *(9)* No wonder they were called "Wow" chips…..

Enough of memory lane. Let's talk about the problem with "low fat". The first dietary guidelines for Americans recommending a low-fat diet were published around 1977. Coincidentally, the obesity epidemic began around the same time. If reduction in fat is because high-fat foods are being replaced with fibrous, unprocessed fruits and vegetables, that is a good thing. But the problem with the "low fat" message as spun by media was/ is this: "The anti-fat message essentially put the blame on saturated fat and cholesterol (harmless), while giving sugar and refined carbs (very unhealthy) a free pass." *(2)* Many, many studies have found it to be " no better at preventing heart disease, obesity or cancer than the standard Western diet." *(2, 10, 11)*

Now, that doesn't mean you should continue with the 'standard Western diet', because the 'standard Western diet' is pretty hideous. No worries, we'll cover how to change that 'standard' diet at the end of this chapter. Once again, processed food causing all sorts of distress on our bodies. The takeaway message from this section: there is plenty of room in your diet for natural, healthy fats.

MODERN WHEAT

Industrialization has brought so many changes to our food supply. What we eat today is so different than the food consumed for the whole history of the human race up until around 100 years ago. Wheat is one of the crops that has changed immensely since the industrialization of farming. In fact, celiac disease (an immune reaction to gluten) has increased four fold in the last half-century alone. Hmmmm....very interesting. Today's 'modern' wheat doesn't even have the same number of chromosomes as ancient wheat varieties do. The oldest wheat in supply today is Einkorn wheat, and it has 14 chromosomes. Modern wheat varieties, and the most common in today's food supply, have between 28 and 42 chromosomes. More chromosomes equals higher levels of gluten. (12) While it has more gluten, it has fewer vital minerals. Levels of magnesium, iron, zinc, and copper are lower in modern wheat varieties. (13) Modern wheat is so different than ancient wheat that many have given it the name "Frankenwheat". Not only does it contain more gluten, but it also contains higher levels of amylopectin A and polypeptides called gluteomorphins. "Say what?", you may be thinking. Well. Amylopectin A is a "super starch" and is really good at making both "Cinnabons and bellies swell". (Just what we need, right?) Then you have gluteomorphins which are polypeptides that have the ability to trigger an opiate-like response in your brain. Nice....this ensures that you will crave more and more Frankenwheat. (14) The fix? Opt for alternative grain products like quinoa, amaranth, millet, and more.

THE "BAD EGG" MISUNDERSTANDING

Much like saturated fats, foods naturally high in cholesterol like eggs have been completely slandered. Despite the fact that studies have failed to show a link between egg consumption and raised bad cholesterol and/or heart disease, eggs still get a bad rap. (13) Our friend the egg needs a public relations makeover. Egg is a good guy. In fact, the protein found in egg whites is considered to be the "perfect protein", and it serves as the standard against which all other proteins are measured. Perfect is in terms of amino acids. A "perfect protein" contains all the essential amino acids. (15) (Quick nutrition lesson/review: amino acids are the building blocks for proteins. The are 20 amino acids. Some are non-essential, which means your body can produce them on its own.

Some are called essential amino acids because your body HAS to obtain these from your diet; it cannot produce them on its own. There are 11 non-essential amino acids and 9 essential amino acids.)

So if you aren't vegan, and you want to chose the best egg, how do you do it? (No Veruca Salt bad eggs!) I am sure by now that you are figuring that pretty much any food considered to be healthy is not processed. But eggs...they just come in a shell....so they should all be the same, right? Sorry, but wrong. You want to choose eggs from organic, pasture-raised hens. Studies have proven them nutritionally superior to eggs from hens raised in cramped chicken houses and fed industrial feed. Pastured eggs have been found to have 1/3 less cholesterol, 1/4 less saturated fat, 2/3 more vitamin A, 2 times more omega-3 fatty acids, 3 times more vitamin E, 7 times more beta carotene and 4 to 6 times the vitamin D of conventional eggs. (16) You know, that whole "you are what you eat" applies to other animals as well. As far as health goes, it matters what you eat whether you are covered in fur or feathers. I should add here that for smaller farming operations, organic certification can be difficult and very expensive to obtain. That being said, you can find high quality eggs that may not bear an organic stamp from your local farmer's market. What to look for? Eggs with bright orange yolks. Such yolks are indicative of hens who have pasture foraged for their vital nutrients. For optimal nutrition, avoid eggs with dull yellow yolks.

ADDITIVES, SYNTHETIC COLORS, & PRESERVATIVES

A big ole' thick book could be written about this section alone. Thousands of additives, synthetic colors, and preservatives exist in our food supply. There is no way to cover all of them in a brief manner, so I will stick to a dirty dozen of them that are BANNED in other countries because they have been deemed unsafe. Remember how we talked about the cocktail effect with EDCs? The same applies for food additives and synthetics. There are many studies which will look at a small amount of a particular additive, then claim it safe. However, the studies which look at such additives in a cocktail manner, which is the way we are exposed to them in real life, have revealed disastrous effects on health. [17]

1. FARM-RAISED SALMON

Farmed and dangerous. Per Jane Houlihan, senior vice president of research for The Environmental Working Group, "Nearly all salmon Americans eat are farm-raised -- grown in dense-packed pens near ocean shores, fed fish meal that can be polluted with toxic PCB chemicals, awash in excrement flushed out to sea and infused with antibiotics to combat unsanitary conditions. Some salmon are raised on farms that use more sustainable methods, but you can't tell from the packaging." [18] Farm-raised salmon contains high levels of PCBs, dioxins and other toxic chemicals. Just as we are what we eat, so are fish. Researchers have found that the source of the contamination for farm-raised salmon is their feed. [19] Their feed is also what gives farm-raised flesh their nice pink color. In the wild, the color comes from a natural compound called astaxanthin. The farm-raised salmon gets its pink color from a synthetic chemical known as carophyll which is manufactured by pharmaceutical giant Hoffman-La Roche. [20] Since consumer reports have shown that people will pay more for redder salmon since it is perceived to be more nutritious, farmers want to color their salmon a nice, deep hue of pink to mimic the actual nutritious, naturally deep pink wild-caught salmon. [21, 22] Therefore, they pump the salmon's fed full of artificial color. Though that farm-raised fish may look similar to its wild-caught cousin, it is lacking in beneficial compounds and full of toxins. Salmon *can* be a very healthy addition to your diet. Opt for wild-caught, not farm-raised.

2. RACTOPAMINE

Ractopamine revs up profits by buffing up lean meat in animals (notably pigs) raised for slaughter. It "raises profits by $2 per head, according to the drug's manufacturer, Elanco, a division of Eli Lilly."

Here we go again with that ching ching of the cash register. Ractopamine works by mimicking stress hormones, making the heart beat faster and relaxing blood vessels, which has led to sickening hundreds of thousands of pigs leaving them too ill to even walk. If you witness a video of this (easily found online), it is disturbing. [23] Since ractopamine is a beta-adrenergic agonist, it isn't classified as a hormone; therefore meat labeled "hormone free" can still contain it. The way to ensure ractopamine-free meat is to buy organic since it is prohibited in organic farming.

3. POTASSIUM BROMATE

Potassium bromate is an additive that is banned in China, Brazil, Canada, the European Union and more, yet totally legal in the United States. Despite its links to cancer, notably thyroid, kidney, and testicular cancers, it has been legal and recognized as safe in the United States since it was patented for baking bread in 1914. [24,25] Potassium bromate is used to bleach flour and to make dough rise faster. California law requires that products containing it must include a warning label. Livescience warns that "Potassium bromate is an unnecessary and potentially harmful food additive, and should be avoided." To avoid it, check the ingredient list for "potassium bromate" or "brominated flour". [24]

4. ARTIFICIAL COLORS

A rainbow of risk. Though they may look pretty, they offer zero nutritional value while posing many health risks. Aaaaand, as usual, it is all in the name of profits. Artificial colors, the majority of which come from petrochemicals like coal and tar, are cheaper to produce than their natural counterparts. Natural colors are anywhere from 8-20 times more expensive than synthetic dyes. All of which really makes me want to say, "Stop the Insanity"! Do we really need the color of our food to be altered anyway? I mean, why can't the green in Kraft's guacamole come from avocados instead of Yellow 5, Yellow 6, and Blue 1? Shouldn't the blue in Aunt Jemima's Blueberry Waffles come from actual blueberries instead of Red 40 and Blue 2? (26) I tried to buy pickles at Target the other day, and I could only find *one* jar out of dozens of brands that did not include artificial food coloring. Despite being linked to allergies, behavioral problems, and cancer, the producers of these dyes do not want things to change because it would bankrupt them. (27)

After all, 15 MILLION pounds of artificial food colors are poured into the US food supply every year. (28) Though plenty of controversy surrounds them, the current FDA approved artificial colors are: FD&C Blue No. 1., FD&C Blue No. 2., FD&C Green No. 3., Orange B., Citrus Red No. 2., FD&C, Red No. 3., FD&C Red No. 40., FD&C Yellow No. 5., and FD&C Yellow No. 6. The list approved for drugs, cosmetics, and medical devices is even longer. (29) True to the reactive rather than proactive nature of public health and wellness, many artificial color additives previously considered safe have be delisted from the FDA's Generally Recognized As Safe (GRAS) list. (FD&C Orange No. 1; FD&C Red No. 32; FD&C Yellows

No. 1, 2, 3, and 4; FD&C Violet No. 1; and FD&C Reds
No. 2 and 4) *(30)* Though evidence continues to mount
against many of the current GRAS colors, stopping the
money train presents a huge challenge. Help the cause by
speaking with your pocketbook. Be a label reader...avoid
buying products with artificial colors. Money talks!
People in other countries have spoken with their wallets.
There are numerous food products that have different
ingredients in the United States versus their overseas
counterparts. *(31)*

5. BROMINATED VEGETABLE OIL (BVO)

You can revisit this little nugget in the previous chapter
about endocrine disrupting chemicals. Basically, this a
flame retardant you can find in your food. It was patented
as a flame retardant for plastics. BVO is used to keep
citrus flavors from separating in sodas and sports drinks.
The FDA first approved this gem...but later changed its
mind and decided that BVO is not so safe after all....but
still allows it to be used as food additive. Go figure.
Health risks associated with BVO include: memory loss,
skin problems and nerve problems. It is banned in Europe
and Japan. *(32)* Avoid BVOs by being a level reader or just
reaching for good ole H2O.

6. SYNTHETIC HORMONES rBGH & rBST

These are synthetic versions of cow hormones used to
increase milk production. Bovine growth hormone (BGH),
also known as *bovine somatotropin* (BST) is the natural
form of this hormone in cattle. The "r" stands for
recombinant and indicates that rBGH and rBST are created
in a lab using genetic engineering. These two were
approved by our dear FDA in 1993. However; their use is

not permitted in the European Union, Canada, and some other countries. Milk from rBGH-treated cows has higher levels of IGF-1, a hormone that normally helps some types of cells to grow. "Several studies have found that IGF-1 levels at the high end of the normal range may influence the development of certain tumors. Some early studies found a relationship between blood levels of IGF-1 and the development of prostate, breast, colorectal, and other cancers." (33) Despite concerns from science-driven data, the FDA continues to claim that rBGH/rBST milk is no different than milk produced from untreated cows. The Ohio court system, however, begs to differ. In 2010 it struck down the FDA's claims of compositionally alike milk citing three major reasons synthetic hormone treated and non-treated milk differs: increased levels of the hormone IGF-1, milk production with lower quality from rBGH/rBST treated cows (higher fat and lower protein), and increased somatic cell counts (meaning more **pus** in the milk because cows treated with synthetic hormones have higher incidence of mastitis). (34) Mmmmmmmm....milk it does a body good....Or does it? With increased growth hormones, more fat, less protein...and my personal favorite....more pus.....I am not so sure processed milk does. Opt for organic milk...rBGH and rBST are prohibited in organic milk production. Even better, reach for organic, grass-fed milk which has a favorable Omega 3 to Omega 6 fatty acid ratio. Or, you could choose a dairy-free option like almond, cashew, or coconut milk. (Check the labels for additives, though. Making your own is another inexpensive option.)

7. AZODICARBONAMIDE (ADA)

Yoga mat in your bread anyone? Used in plastic and rubber products like yoga mats and flip flops, to make them softer and more stretchy; this marvel is also used in bread, bagels, pastries, pizza, tortillas, hamburger and hot dog buns to bleach flour, and to make dough more elastic. It is used by more than 130 companies including but not limited to: Betty Crocker, Pillsbury, Little Debbie, Earth Grains, Artisan's Choice, Starbuck's, Marie Callendar's, McDonald's, Burger King, Wendy's, Arby's, Dunkin Donuts, and more. *(35)* So why should you be concerned that ADA is lurking in so many processed foods? It has been linked to both asthma and skin allergies. *(36)* Nip it and other processed foods from your diet, and you may find yourself feeling better and better. (Though the efffff-deee-A may get torn up for anyone suggesting an approach as crazy as food quality being linked to your health.)

8. BHA and BHT

I'll just quote LiveScience on this one: "Here's a question for you: What food additive does the Food and Drug Administration deem "generally recognized as safe," while the National Institutes of Health, says it's "reasonably anticipated to be a human carcinogen?" Here's a hint: It's a preservative, and you can find it in (drum roll, please): potato chips, lard, butter, cereal, instant mashed potatoes, preserved meat, beer, baked goods, dry beverage and dessert mixes, chewing gum, and other foods. Oh, also: rubber, petroleum products, and, of course, wax food packaging." And the answer: BHA and its first cousin BHT *(37)* These are used as preservatives…but vitamin E can serve the same purpose naturally. Yet again my friends, check food labels. Avoid BHA and BHT

9. CARRAGEENAN

In the list of additives, this one is the black sheep because it is *not synthetic*. Though it is *natural*, it definitely poses health risks. With most of the additives we've been discussing, you can simply opt for products labeled "organic" and you are good to go. But since carrageenan is derived from a natural source (red algae), it is allowed under organic guidelines. The purpose of carrageenan is to keep the ingredients in liquids and foods like yogurt well mixed. (The addition of carrageenan could be avoided by simply adding a "Shake Well" label to such products.) You also find carrageenan in lunch meats, even the organic ones.

So why is natural carrageenan bad? It causes your digestive tract to act much in the same way it does as when it is invaded by Salmonella. Joanne Tobacman, MD, associate professor of clinical medicine at the University of Illinois School of Medicine at Chicago explains that carrageenan predictably causes inflammation which leads to ulcerations and even bleeding. Dr. Tobacman's research in lab animals has linked carrageenan to gastrointestinal cancer, diabetes, and ulcerative colitis. Scan labels for foods that contain carrageenan, as it can be present in organic brands. The good news is that many organics companies, including Stonyfield Farm, So Delicious, Eden Foods, and Oregon Ice Cream, are voluntarily working to remove carrageenan from their products. *(38)*

10. ANTIBIOTIC INFUSED MEAT

Yikes. This one causes a complex web of problems. "Every time antibiotics are used in any setting, bacteria evolve by developing resistance. This process can happen with alarming speed," said Steve Solomon, M.D., director of CDC's Office of Antimicrobial Resistance. "These drugs are a precious, limited resource—the more we use antibiotics today, the less likely we are to have effective antibiotics tomorrow." (39)

While there has definitely been a problem in recent years with over-prescription of antibiotics for humans, most antibiotics are actually used in animal agriculture. 13.1 million kilograms of antibacterial drugs were sold for use on animals in 2009 which accounted for around 74% of all antibiotics used in the United States that year. (40,41) That's an enormous amount of antibiotics! Such overuse of antibiotics has lead to the evolution of some exceptionally scary antibiotic-resistant superbugs. The CDC reports that these superbugs are responsible for more than TWO MILLION illnesses per year and TWENTY THREE THOUSAND deaths. (These numbers do not include an additional 250,000 illnesses and 14,000 deaths due to *Clostridium difficile. C. diff* is directly related to antibiotic use and resistance.)

Both overprescription *and* overuse of antibiotics have been problems in recent years. People go to the doctor and don't feel like they've been treated unless they leave with a z-pack or other antibiotic. Never mind that antibiotics do zilch for viruses. Never mind that they are sometimes prescribed 'just in case'. Never mind that they may be doing your body more harm than good if you take them when they aren't truly needed. Never mind all of that...people just want their prescriptions! The Centers for Disease Control addresses this by saying, "The loss of effective antibiotic treatments will also undermine treatment of infectious complications in patients with other diseases. Many medical advances—joint replacements, organ transplants, cancer therapy, rheumatoid arthritis therapy – are dependent on the ability to fight infections with antibiotics. If the ability to effectively treat those infections is lost, the ability to safely offer people many of the life-saving and life-improving modern medical advances will be lost with it." (39)

Antibiotics certainly saved my life during cancer treatment when I was faced more than once with life-threatening bacterial infections. So, I am not trying to vilify antibiotics. Antibiotics when used properly are miracles! The problem is the *overuse* of them.

Overprescription in doctors' offices and overuse by humans is a big piece of the puzzle. However, I'd venture to say that overuse in the agricultural industry is an even bigger problem considering that the antibiotics used for livestock account for around three fourths of all antibiotics used in the United States.

It was not always this way.

How did we get here? Well, well, well…guess what…we are going on another trip down the money trail. No surprise there. Let's travel back to 1948 when antibiotics were new on the scene. That year, biochemist Thomas H. Jukes and his team at Lederle Laboratories were working on an antibiotic known as Aureomycin. Of course there were high hopes that Aureomycin would be a lifesaving drug, but the scientists also hoped to find another way to rake in profits from it. During Aureomycin research Mr. Jukes discovered that when added to chick-feed, it greatly boosted chicks' growth. (42) Some chicks even grew to weigh twice as much as those in the control group. (43) Knowing this, Jukes wanted to do more studies. However, his bosses cut off his supply of Aureomycin due to human demand. Not one to be deterred, Jukes dug through the lab's trash to find leftovers from the production of the antibiotic. "Trash, it turned out, could be transformed into meat" and profits. Cha-Ching! Research at the time showed that not only farm animals got fatter and bigger with habitual antibiotic use, but that humans did too.

Alexander Fleming, the discoverer of penicillin, warned that making people larger with antibiotics may do more harm than good. But this was America in an era when bigger was viewed as better. And so the antibiotic-from-garbage-laced feed became ubiquitous on American farms. "The drug-laced feeds allowed farmers to keep their animals indoors — because in addition to becoming meatier, the animals now could subsist in filthy conditions. The stage was set for the factory farm." (43)

Well then. Isn't that lovely. Overuse of antibiotics on farms is creating superbugs *and* making us fat.

To avoid antibiotics in your meat, choose organic.

11. PHOSPHATE ADDITIVES

Phosphates are added to processed foods for a variety of reasons. They may serve as emulsifiers, as texturizing agents, as leavening agents, or as neutralizing agents. (44) Phosphate additives are bad, bad, bad for your arteries. They are considered arterial toxins and can cause your arteries to stiffen within hours of consumption. (45) They cause damage by endothelial dysfunction and vascular calcification. (46) "Recently, a high-normal serum phosphate concentration has also been found to be an independent predictor of cardiovascular events and mortality in the general population....the public should be informed that added phosphate is damaging to health." (45) Besides wreaking havoc on your arteries, phosphate additives also do a number on your bones. All of that phosphate disrupts the proper ratio of calcium to phosphorus leading to less bone density and weakened bones. *(47)*

Now, we do need phosphorus in our bodies....but it should come from natural sources. Organic phosphates found naturally in foods are absorbed differently than synthetic phosphate additives. Sodas are a HUGE source of phosphate additives. Packaged, non-organic meats and fast food are also full of phosphate additives, so take care to avoid them.

12. GMOs

Though GMOs are not technically additives or preservatives, they are so bad, bad, very bad that they earned a whole separate category in this chapter. Read all about them in the next section.

GMOs

(This one is a huge soapbox issue for me, so get ready!)

A GMO (Genetically Modified Organism) is an organism whose genetic material has been altered using genetic engineering techniques. **This is not traditional crossbreeding and cannot occur in nature.** Genetically modifying is altering the DNA of a plant to produce a trait that is *not natural* in the *species*. The DNA comes from things like *viruses* and *bacteria*. Crops are engineered with the intent to be resistant to other viruses or bacteria, resistant to herbicides or pesticides, have altered starch or fat content, and/ or more.

Though a genetically modified fruit or veggie may look the same, so buyer beware. An ear of corn by any name may taste quite sweet, but those little GMO frankenkernals of corn may jump right off the cob and bite you back. Figuratively, at least. Odds are, you are eating the frankenfoods all the time while blissfully unaware since the labeling of GMO foods and ingredients is not required in the United States. There are no restrictions against GMOs in the US; however, most developed nations do not consider GMOs to be safe. In more than 60 countries around the world there are significant restrictions or outright bans on the production and sale of GMOs.

Before we talk about all the reasons GMOs are bad for you, let's first talk about who brought them into existence and the REAL reasons why. If you want the short and sweet answer, two words really sum it up: Monsanto and Money. Seems you can always find your answer if you follow the money trail. Let's look at a brief history of the Monsanto company. Their history alone is enough to make me know that I do not want them anywhere near my food supply.

Created in 1901, Monsanto first produced the artificial sweetener saccharin.(48) Saccharin has no nutritional value, and it has been linked to cancer, diabetes, allergic reaction, and weight gain.(49) In 1917 they began producing aspirin.(50) By the 1920s, they had expanded their production into basic industrial chemicals. Monsanto continued to gobble up other companies and added soaps, detergents, synthetic rubber, plastics, and more to their list. Next they added uranium research for the Manhattan Project during World War II. (If your history is rusty, Manhattan Project equals atomic bomb.) (48) The 40s brought the addition of polystyrene production. Polystyrene poses numerous environmental and health risks including neurological disfunction and cancer. (51) Ok- so we aren't even 100 years into Monsanto's history, and you are probably wondering how a chemical/nuclear/plastics company got involved in the food business. More importantly, you may be wondering what in the hell makes it ok for a chemical/nuclear/plastics company to be in control of the food you eat.

Prezactly, people. Prezactly.

Keep reading, because it gets even better!

Enter agrochemicals and enormous profits. After the second World War, Monsanto began churning out chemical pesticides and herbicides including 2,4,5-T, DDT, Lasso and Agent Orange (a mixture of half 2,4,5-T and half 2,4 D) . Health risks associated with 2,4,5-T include cough, sore throat, diarrhea, drowsiness, headache, nausea, vomiting, and cancer. Additionally, it is classified as an endocrine disruptor. *(52)* DDT was so horrible that it is no longer in production. It can still be found in our soil and food supply.....and it was banned in 1972! Banned over 45 years ago, and it is still causing problems. Harmful effects include: cancer, liver damage, nervous system damage, and damage to the reproductive system. *(53)* Then we have Agent Orange, which was used as a defoliant in the Vietnam War. It contaminated more than 3,000,000 civilians and servicemen. An estimated 500,000 Vietnamese children have been born with deformities attributed to it. Half a million. *(48)* While Monsanto was raking it in overseas with Agent Orange, they were making big bucks at home with the herbicide Lasso which they began producing in 1969.   Continuing to expand their agriculture division, Monsanto began producing Roundup (active ingredient glyphosate) in 1976. Studies have found glyphosate to be "insidious" and slowly manifesting causing inflammation which "damages cellular systems throughout the body" leading to a host of health problems like Parkinson's disease, infertility, and cancer. *(54)*

Bear with me, I promise we are getting close to the GMO part, but let's pause for just a minute to talk more about Monsanto's history since the 1970s and some of the lawsuits against them (and at the time of print, there are thousands of pending lawsuits against the company):

- "1986--Monsanto found guilty of negligently exposing a worker to benzene at its Chocolate Bayou Plant in Texas. It is forced to pay $100 million to the family of Wilbur Jack

Skeen, a worker who died of leukemia after repeated exposures."

- "1987--Monsanto is one of the companies named in an $180 million settlement for Vietnam War veterans exposed to Agent Orange."
- "1988--A federal jury finds Monsanto Co.'s subsidiary, G.D. Searle & Co., negligent in testing and marketing of its Copper 7 intrauterine birth control device (IUD)." The device caused pelvic inflammations, ectopic pregnancies or perforation of the uterus, and sometimes resulted in infertility. "The verdict followed the *unsealing of internal documents* regarding safety concerns about the IUD, which was used by nearly 10 million women between 1974 and 1986." The sealed *internal* documents show that Monsanto was well aware of the dangers of its IUD.
- "1990--EPA chemists allege fraud in Monsanto's 1979 dioxin study, which found exposure to the chemical doesn't increase cancer risks"
- "1990--Monsanto spends more than $405,000 to defeat California's pesticide regulation Proposition 128, known as the "Big Green" initiative. The initiative is aimed at phasing out the use of pesticides, including Monsanto's product alachlor, linked to cancer"
- "1991--Monsanto is fined $1.2 million for trying to conceal discharge of contaminated waste water into the Mystic River in Connecticut."
- 1993 — Creates synthetic hormones rBGH and rBST (brand name Posilac) to stimulate greater milk production in cows.
- "1995--Monsanto is sued after allegedly supplying radioactive material for a controversial study which involved feeding radioactive iron to 829 pregnant women."
- "1995--Monsanto ordered to pay $41.1 million to a waste management company in Texas due to concerns over hazardous waste dumping." (48)

- Early 2000s…this one happened in Anniston, Alabama which is just down the road from my hometown of Gadsden. For years, Monsanto had produced PCBs (polychlorinated biphenyls) and dumped toxic wastes in Anniston. (Remember PCBs from the previous chapter…they are heinous and considered to be one of the most serious and troubling chemical threats to our planet. The EPA says that they have been demonstrated to cause cancer, as well as a variety of other adverse health effects on the immune system, reproductive system, nervous, and endocrine systems. Yikes.) *So for 40 years,* Monsanto literally dumped poison into the creeks of Anniston. According to an article written by the Washington post, thousands of documents marked "CONFIDENTIAL: Read and Destroy" were uncovered showing that Monsanto knew exactly what they were doing, but kept doing it in the name of profits. (See a trend here? Time and time again it has been shown that Monsanto has knowingly caused harm and covered it up.) Get this: "In **1966**, Monsanto managers discovered that fish submerged in that creek turned belly-up within 10 seconds, spurting blood and shedding skin as if dunked into boiling water. They told no one. In 1969, they found fish in another creek with 7,500 times the legal PCB levels. They decided "there is little object in going to expensive extremes in limiting discharges." In 1975, a company study found that PCBs caused tumors in rats. They ordered its conclusion changed from "slightly tumorigenic" to "does not appear to be carcinogenic." Makes me nauseated to even think about it. Further, "We can't afford to lose one dollar of business," one internal memo concluded.". *(55)* Bastards. Can't afford to lose a dollar of business, but they can poison others in the name of money. So. Very. Repugnant. But wait…this particular case gets even better….knowing they were caught on the carpet….they managed to divert this division to a new company called Solutia so that when they were eventually

169

ordered to pay 600 million dollars in claims settlements and billions in environmental cleanup, all that Solutia had to do was file for Chapter 11 Bankruptcy to squirm out of it. (48)

- 2018 - - Jurors give $289 million to a man who developed cancer from Monsanto's Roundup weedkiller. (103)

How do these people sleep at night, and where in the world is Erin Brokovich? We need you on this one, sister!

Okay, okay, back to Monsanto and the GMOs. By the late 1980s and the early 1990s, the Roundup weedkiller contributed to about 20% of sales and around 45% of operating income for Monsanto. Even today, glyphosate (the active ingredient in Roundup) remains the world's biggest herbicide by volume of sales.

Cash. Cow.

With knowledge that the patents protecting its monopoly on glyphosate would be expiring in they year 2000, Monsanto needed to come up with a plan to prolong the life of glyphosate and keep them filthy rich. Now....we are finally getting to the GMO part. Enter "Roundup Ready" seeds. Basically, this meant that farmers could spray glyphosate (which we've already established to be revolting) all over their fields to kill everything except their chosen crop. Their public relations spin was that they would create nutritionally superior crops with increased yields so that they could feed the world.

Mmmmhhhhmmmmm. Not buying it.

All you have to do is read the report "Failure to Yield" to realize this is a lie. (56) So now Monsanto would make a bajillion dollars on selling seeds they had the patents for and another bajillion dollars on extra Roundup sales. How convenient. They patent seeds that will require millions of pounds of their very own poisonous glyphosate. Brilliant in the most evil way.

In the years since the first GMO crops hit the market in 1996, there has been a glyphosate geyser. Partly due to the fact that more and more GMO crops have been planted, and partly due to the fact that over time and overuse of Roundup has created resistant superweeds, thus calling for more and more Roundup to be used. So, on top of the massive amounts of Roundup sold by Monsanto, they have also attempted to monopolize their GMO seeds. By 2007, NINETY PERCENT of the world area devoted to GM crops were from Monsanto seeds and traits. Additionally, they devote an annual budget of 10 million dollars to "harassing, intimidating, suing, and in some cases bankrupting American farmers over alleged improper use of its patented seeds." (48) Ummmmm....scary.

Basically, I have one word for Monsanto: **Devil**. If those few paragraphs aren't enough alone to convince you that you don't wan't Monsanto anywhere near your food, you can keep reading for examples of why GMOs are both bad for your health and the health of the planet.

Why are GMOs bad? Let's start with the fact that they are simply unhealthy. The American Academy of Environmental Medicine (AAEM) urges doctors to prescribe non-GMO diets for all patients. The AAEM says:

> "Because GM foods pose a serious health risk in the areas of toxicology, allergy and immune function, reproductive health, and metabolic, physiologic and genetic health and are without benefit".

The AAEM advises us to not wait before even more evidence mounts against the deleterious effects of GMOs. Specially, they looked at many different studies and found that:

> "Multiple animal studies show significant immune dysregulation, including up-regulation of cytokines associated with asthma, allergy, and inflammation. Animal studies also show altered structure and function of the liver, including altered lipid and carbohydrate metabolism as well as cellular changes that could lead to accelerated aging and possibly lead to the accumulation of reactive oxygen species (ROS). Changes in the

kidney, pancreas and spleen have also been documented. A recent 2008 study links GM corn with infertility, showing a significant decrease in offspring over time and significantly lower litter weight in mice fed GM corn. This study also found that over 400 genes were found to be expressed differently in the mice fed GM corn. These are genes known to control protein synthesis and modification, cell signaling, cholesterol synthesis, and insulin regulation. Studies also show intestinal damage in animals fed GM foods, including proliferative cell growth and disruption of the intestinal immune system."

(57)

Moreover, since the debut of GMOs in 1996, the percentage of Americans with three or more chronic illnesses jumped from 7% to 13% in just 9 years; food allergies skyrocketed, and disorders such as autism, reproductive disorders, digestive problems, and others are on the rise. *(58)*

Once you go 'whack' with the DNA, you can't go back. Therefore, GMOs contaminate FOREVER. (Remember that to produce a GMO, genes are removed from other species like viruses and bacteria and then they are inserted into chosen seeds, thus changing their genetic makeup.) Once planted, GMO species can cross pollinate and their seeds can travel. It is impossible to fully clean up our contaminated gene pool. *(58)* It has been found that our traditional seed supply has already been contaminated with DNA from genetically engineered crops. *(59)*

Once DNA is changed, it is a done deal. Permanent. The very blueprint of life rewritten. Additionally, GMO contamination has also caused economic losses for organic and non-GMO farmers who often struggle to keep their crops pure.

The eternal contamination is not limited to plant environments. Here is where it gets even scarier. One type of GM crop involves the insertion of genes from the Bt (*Bacillus thuringiensis*) bacterium. Once insects ingest these Bt genes, holes form in their digestive system thereby poisoning and killing them. Bt crops are touted as being insect resistant.

But what happens when WE eat those crops designed to produce holes in the digestive system of insects?

Human studies have shown how such genetically modified (GM) food can leave material behind inside us, possibly causing long-term problems. (60) The toxic insecticide produced by GM corn was found in the blood of pregnant women and their unborn babies. (58) This toxin wreaks havoc on the intestinal flora and digestive system, and since "cross discipline research shows a correlation between gut health and autism" there is reason to suspect GMOs are causing the rise in autism we are seeing in this country. Twenty years ago, autism was rare. In 2008, 1 in 54 boys were diagnosed with an autism spectrum disorder(ASD), and those with an ASD have a disproportionately high level of digestive problems including inflammation and leaky gut. Additionally, "numerous healthcare practitioners report greater success when they address the gastrointestinal disorder as part of their autism treatment protocol". (60) Beyond autism, leaky gut syndrome is linked to atherosclerosis, congestive heart failure, cancer, depression, liver disease and more. (61,62,63)

Even the American Academy of Pediatrics warns against them stating that "Epidemiologic evidence demonstrates associations between early life exposure to pesticides and pediatric cancers, decreased cognitive function, and behavioral problems". They explain that the risks are both acute and chronic. (64)

GMOs increase herbicide use. Between 1996 and 2008, US farmers sprayed an extra 383 million pounds of herbicide on GMOs. (58) That is a lot of poison, y'all. With all that increase in dangerous glyphosate, Monsanto has managed to create an environment for superweeds which are now resistant to their golden egg glyphosate/Roundup. And would you know that because of all those superweeds created by GMOs and the overuse of glyphosate, the FDA has recently approved the use of 2,4 D for use on GMO crops. (65) Well, well, well.....if you are already thinking that 2,4 D sounds familiar but you can't remember why....just back up a few paragraphs....it makes up half of the deadly duo in *Agent Orange*.

The damage doesn't stop with humans, either. GMO crops and the herbicides and pesticides associated with them harm the environment. Let's not forget about our furry, feathered, and scaly friends They are harmed as well. Biodiversity is reduced. Water and soil pollution occur causing ecosystems to become unsustainable. *(58)*

What about those Monsanto promises about ending world hunger and such?

GMOs, on average, do not increase yields. Both the Union of Concerned Scientists' 2009 report "Failure to Yield" and The International Assessment of Agricultural Knowledge, Science and Technology for Development (IAASTD) report, *authored by more than 400 scientists and backed by 58 governments found this.* The latter report states that GM crop yields were "highly variable" and in some cases, "yields declined." *(66, 56)*

How is all of this possible???

"Money! It's a gas. Grab that cash with both hands and make a stash. New car, caviar, four star daydream, think I'll buy a football team" - Pink Floyd.

So we have money. Then inextricably linked is the the government's downright negligent oversight on the manner. Enter the US Food and Drug Administration (FDA). They do not require any labeling of GMO products. Monsanto has spent MASSIVE amounts of money to lobby against any state laws that would require labeling of foods containing GMOs. They do not even want people to be aware when they are buying their frankenfoods out of fear that consumers, when given the choice, may opt to purchase something else. Monsanto recently spent $46 million, yes...FORTY SIX MILLION DOLLARS...on the "No on 37" campaign in California. Proposition 37 would have made GMO labeling mandatory in California. *Note that I didn't say that Prop 37 would have outlawed GMOs, it would have simply required labeling so that consumers could decide whether or not to purchase them*. Apparently their **$46 million** spent in an effort to dupe the masses worked as Prop 37 did not pass....it slipped by with a narrow margin of 53 to 47 percent. (If a company has *forty six million dollars* to spend on a campaign to block labeling of their GMOs, how much profit do you think they are raking in year after year?)(67)

Propositions to label aren't just happening in California, so I urge you to please vote to label should it come to a vote in your state. Eventually, Monsanto's public relations budget for propaganda has to run thin.

Now back to the FDA. It does not require companies to even notify them before putting GMO foods on the market. The FDA and Monsanto are really cozy. The FDA's food czar, Michael Taylor, was once Monsanto's lawyer and later their vice president. I smell a rat....do you? Finally, when a public lawsuit showed an overwhelming consensus that GMOs can "create unpredictable, hard-to-detect side effects", long term safety studies were recommended. Alas, the White House instead urged the FDA to promote biotechnology and the official agency in charge of that policy was none other than Michael Taylor. (58) He spent several decades shuffling between Monsanto, the FDA, and the USDA. Conflict of interest much?

Oy ve! What to do?

Avoid GMOs like the plague. Don't buy them! Nothing speaks louder than dollars spent, or rather...not spent. By avoiding purchase of GMOs, you contribute to consumer rejection. With enough rejection, GMO ingredients will become a marketing liability, and food companies will give them the boot.

How do you avoid them? It is easier than you think. Most processed foods contain GMOs, so buy as little of them as possible. Which is a win/win, because nothing healthy comes from processed junk anyway. Top GMO foods include: soy (in tons of processed foods in the form of soy protein, soybean oil, etc), corn (again, in tons of processed foods: cornstarch, corn syrup, etc) sugar beets (ummm....refined sugar....again in processed foods), canola, alfalfa, cotton, milk, sugar, aspartame, tomatoes, zucchini, yellow squash, and papaya. Look for foods that are certified organic or that bear the Non-GMO project seal. Organic foods cannot contain GMOs. So if it is labeled organic, it should be GMO free. There are some foods which are not organic, but that bear the Non-GMO project emblem.

THE GOOD

Whew! I know I just blew it up with a lot of information on the 'bad'. As with any situation, I like to get the bad out of the way first so that I can finish on a good note. Once upon a time, ALL food was organic, grass-fed, and unprocessed. Agriculture was a regenerative process. Consumer demand has been driving an increase in organically produced foods since the 1990s. In fact, organically produced goods have shown a double-digit increase most years since 1990. *(68)*

If you ask me, that is GREAT news. It means that more and more consumers understand the importance of avoiding harmful chemicals and additives. It means that such consumers are growing in numbers and their collective voices are speaking loudly. It makes me happy. I hope the information in this chapter thus far has opened your eyes and inspired you to devote time and energy into nixing the bad in your diet and replacing it with good, nourishing foods.

We spent a lot of time talking about the bad things in food....all the things that can act as slow poisons over time. Time to talk about the *good*. The ways food can *nourish* and *sustain* us. Make us more energetic and less lethargic. Improve our skin. Decrease our risks for cancer and autoimmune diseases. Help our immune systems function more effectively and efficiently. The body has an incredible ability to restore itself when given the right environment to do it.

THE SHORT VERSION

Avoid processed foods. Eat dense nutrition. (That'd be foods that provide numerous nutrients for a relatively small number of calories.) Eat a variety of foods.

THE LONGER VERSION

Highlighted below are some of the best foods in the whole wide world. They all have proven anti-cancer properties. An anti-cancer diet is a great way to eat no matter what. Such a diet is beneficial in preventing heart disease, cancer, auto-immune diseases and more. When the right portions are chosen, it is highly unlikely that you'll be fat while very likely that you will feel full of energy.

Cruciferous Veggies

In terms of dense nutrition, I'd say this group is a flat out bunch of SUPERSTARS. No other group as a whole is higher in concentrations of Vitamin A carotenoids, Vitamin C, folic acid and fiber. Also rich in manganese and Vitamin K, along with generous amounts of protein, calcium, Omega 3 fatty acids, and numerous phytonutrients, cruciferous veggies should be considered the most splendid vegetable stars in the galaxy. When you have a food that is rich in vitamins, minerals, macronutrients (fats, proteins, or carbohydrates), phytonutrients (natural micronutrients occurring in plants....more than 25,000 have been identified), and fiber for a small amount of calories, you've got yourself a winner.

Cruciferous veggies are sometimes also called cruciform, brassica, or mustard family vegetables. You may hear farmers referring to them as "cole crops". Hence the reason certain cabbage and broccoli dishes are called coleslaw. Cruciferous vegetables include: arugula, broccoli, brussels sprouts, cabbage, cauliflower, Chinese cabbage (napa cabbage and bok choy), collard greens, daikon radish, horseradish, kale, kohlrabi, land cress, mustard greens, radish, rutabaga, shepherd's purse, turnip, and watercress.

Studies have shown that the bioavailability of beta-carotene, lutein, and retinol from cruciferous veggies to be extremely impressive. In the studies, people who consumed a generous portion during a meal showed significant increases in the blood levels of such antioxidant nutrients. Vitamin K (kale and collards have especially high concentrations) has been shown to clearly regulate our inflammatory response. If your body is in a constant state of inflammation, bad things from allergies and arthritis to fibromyalgia, heart disease and cancer can result. By regulating inflammation, Vitamin K can reduce chronic inflammation thereby reducing your risk for a host of maladies.

When considering nutrients like fiber, protein, calcium, and omega 3 fatty acids, many equate the source with things like grains, meat, dairy, and fish. So many seem to be unaware that you can get all of these winners through vegetables….especially our cruciferous superstars. Just 200 calories of broccoli provides 20 grams of protein. Two hundred calories of cruciferous veggies can provide from 50-80% of your daily fiber requirement! Two hundred calories of kale provides you with half your daily recommended value of calcium. That same 200 calories of cruciferous vegetables provides somewhere between around 600 and 1000 milligrams of omega 3 fatty acid.

Of all the goodness we've just discussed, we haven't even begun to talk about phytonutrients. Notable phytonutrients in cruciferous veggies belong to a group known as glucosinolates which have a great track record for reducing cancer risk. The glucosinolates in cruciferous vegetables with known health benefits include: erucin, glucoallyn, glucobrassicanapin, gluconapin, gluconasturtin, glucophanin, iberin, progoitrin, sinigrin, 4-methyloxyglucobrassicin. Don't worry- you don't have to be able to pronounce them to get the health benefits! (69)

Cruciferous veggies also contain sulforaphane and indole-3 carbinols (I3cs). These are powerfully anti-cancer because they have the ability to detoxify certain carcinogenic substances. They have been shown to prevent precancerous cells from developing into malignant tumors. They promote cancer cell apoptosis (cancer cell death) and they block angiogenesis (the formation of a new blood supply to feed a tumor). (17)

So we've established that cruciferous veggies to be spectacular, but how to prepare? If "To cook or not to cook is the question", "Both" is the answer! Make a smoothie or a salad…dip 'em in some hummus…steam them, put them in some soup, or stir-fry them. Recent research shows there is a beneficial place for cruciferous vegetables in both raw and cooked form. In the raw form, nutrients from cruciferous veggies are more likely to be absorbed in the upper digestive tract and transported to the liver where they are made available to other tissues in the body. When eating raw, opt for the freshest available. Freshly picked veggies (less than 48 hours) have the most active enzymes. Freshly chopped and cooked cruciferous veggies are more likely to pass through the upper digestive tract unabsorbed to the lower digestive tract (colon). At this point they are likely further metabolized by bacteria in the colon which may account for the risk reduction of colon cancer seen for the intake of cruciferous veggies. The one method of cooking that *isn't* recommend if you want to get optimal health benefits is boiling which can destroy sulflorophane and I3Cs. *(17)*

One more thing that makes the cruciferous food group special is that we typically consume many different parts of the plant. Flowers: broccoli florets….leaves: mustard, collard, & turnip greens; kale; etc…stems and stalks: broccoli…roots: turnips, rutabagas, radishes….seeds: mustard. Plants store their phytonutrients in different anatomical parts, so the fact that we eat so many parts of cruciferous plants is uniquely positive. (69)

So get busy eating your cruciferous veggies. They certainly do a body good!

Carotenoid-rich Veggies and Fruits

When you think of carotenoid-rich vegetables and fruits, think of yellows, oranges, and reds (though some dark green veggies fall in this category, too). This group includes things like carrots, yams, sweet potatoes, squash, guava, watermelon, papaya, red peppers pumpkins, tomatoes, persimmons, apricots, beets, and so forth. I'd venture to say the most widely-known nutrient supplied by this bunch is Vitamin A, so we'll start there. Vitamin A enters your body in different forms and is then converted into various usable forms. Carotenoids serve as most of the world's Vitamin A source. It is necessary for proper functioning of the retina in the eye, for growth and development of skeletal and soft tissues, and it plays a role in iron metabolism. Vitamin A, especially in the form of beta-carotene and other carotenoids, is an extremely important antioxidant. You often hear about the benefits of antioxidants, but maybe you can't really explain why they are beneficial. Think of it like this: Our environment exposes us to all sorts of free radicals. A free radical is any atom or molecule that has a single unpaired electron in an outer shell. I know you don't want a chemistry lesson, but this one is short…promise! Electrons hate feeling lonely. They do not like to be single. They'll do anything to make a pair. They will attack and attach themselves to cellular structures in your body thus causing damage. This is where antioxidants are helpful. Antioxidants will seek out those free radicals and pair with them before they attack your body. Essentially, they take one for the team. From a cancer standpoint, this is awesome because the damage from the oxidation of cells (from things like free radicals) impairs the body's defense against some cancers. So, a healthy supply of antioxidants is helpful in protecting against cancer. (70) And if cancer has already struck, they are helpful in helping to fight it. "A study that tracked breast cancer patients for 6 years showed that those who consumed the most carotenoids lived longer than those who consumed less." *(17)*

Another key nutrient found in carotenoid-rich foods is lycopene. It stimulates the growth of immune cells, and it has been concluded to contribute to longer survival rates in prostate cancer patients. For lycopene to be bioavailable, it should be cooked. Lycopene, lutein, phytoene, and canthaxanthin (phytonutrients also found in carotenoid-rich foods) increase immune cells' ability to attack tumor cells. Additionally, these nutrients make NK cells more aggressive. (NK= Natural Killer cells...a type of white blood cell playing a major role in attacking both viruses and tumors.) *(17)*

It is important to note that it is best to get nutrients from food or whole food supplements versus taking synthetic supplements. Lycopene is a great example. Tomatoes contain a whole series of anticancer nutrients whose *combined* action is more effective than lycopene on its own. *(17)* Since Vitamin A is one of the fat-soluble vitamins (meaning your body stores excess rather than excreting it readily), taking too much of a synthetic supplement can lead to toxicity. But "toxicity studies in animals have shown that beta-carotene is not carcinogenic, mutagenic, or teratogenic." *(70)* This means that tons of beta-carotene from plant sources won't cause cancer, mutations, or birth defects. The worst thing that can happen is that your skin may turn an orangey/yellow color. (Anyone who's ever fed their baby too many sweet potatoes has probably witnessed this!) When excess intakes are curbed, the skin clears in a relatively short time. Mother Nature really does know best! She's been doing her thing for quite some time now.

Berries

Strawberries, blackberries, raspberries, cranberries...you know, pretty much anything that ends in "berry". These all contain high amounts of ellagic acid and polyphenols, both of which help detoxify carcinogens and inhibit angiogenesis. *(17)* Ellagic acid has been shown to cause cancer cell apoptosis (death) in human bladder cancer cell lines in addition to having strong anti-proliferative activity against the colon, breast, and prostatic cancer cell lines investigated. *(71) (72)* As for polyphenols, their benefits are extensive. Polyphenols have shown the ability to "scavenge the free radicals formed during the pathological process like cancer, cardiovascular diseases and neurodegenerative disorders". Additionally, recent research is showing promise for using dietary polyphenols in the treatment of Alzheimer's disease. *(73)* Berries are also great in the fight against osteoporosis.

There are many ways to enjoy berries. I most often eat them big-bowl-o-fruit style or smoothie style.....probably because these are the two simplest ways to consume them. My freezer stays stocked with frozen organic fruit. All you have to do is toss some in a good blender, add a splash of water and blend away. (I also throw in some chia seeds for fiber, protein, and omega 3 fatty acids.) "Fast food" at its finest. No need to worry that frozen fruits are any less nutritious. Freezing does not harm the anticancer molecules found in such fruits. *(17)*

Stone Fruits

This group contains fruits like peaches, mangoes, apricots, cherries, and plums. Just think about fruits that have a pit. Recent research has shown that stone fruits have just as many cancer fighting agents as berries, but typically at a much lower cost. *(17)* Again, I find myself usually enjoying these fruits plain and simple or in a frozen smoothie. Easy breezy. Are you noticing a trend? No where in the list of healthy and cancer-fighting foods will you find processed or drive-through selections.

Citrus Fruits

The benefits of citrus fruits like oranges, tangerines, lemons, limes, and grapefruit are numerous. Citrus fruits are high in flavonoids. Remember when we talked about polyphenols in the berry section? Flavonoids actually belong in the polyphenol family, and they are best known for their antioxidant and anti-inflammatory health benefits. They support healthy cardiovascular and nervous systems. They have also been associated with a deceased risk of both lung and breast cancers, since they stimulate the detoxification of certain carcinogens. (17,74) The specific flavonoids tangeritin and nobiletin, found in the rinds of tangerines, have been shown to be effective against both brain cancer cells and breast cancer cells. (75,76) Naringenin, a phytonutrient mainly present in citrus fruits and tomatoes, has gained increasing interest because of its positive health effects not only in cancer prevention but also in non-cancer diseases. (77) Citrus aurantifolia from lime peels has recently been shown to increase the effectiveness of chemotherapeutic drugs against breast cancer cells. (78) I could go on and on with more studies. The thing that is promising to me, is that more and more RECENT research is highlighting different phytonutrients. Though big pharma would not like us to believe it, more evidence is being built that nutrition certainly matters when it comes to cancer….and good health. So, grab a tangerine, and keep on reading!

Olives/Olive Oil

The word on the street for many years has been that there isn't a diet much healthier than a Mediterranean style diet. Known for promoting lifelong health, the Mediterranean diet consists mainly of fruits and vegetables, beans and nuts, healthy grains, fish, olive oil, small amounts of dairy, and red wine. Olives and olive oil play a key role in the Mediterranean diet. They are good sources of antioxidants known as phenols, which are excellent at both supporting heart health and kicking cancer cells. A recent study which looked at the biological activities of the particular polyphenol oleuropein, the most prevalent polyphenol present in olives, found it to have antioxidant, anti-inflammatory, anti-tumor, hepatoprotective (protects your liver) and antimicrobial effects. No wonder it has been used through the ages in natural remedies to treat numerous conditions. *(79)* Extra-virgin olive oil (EVOO) derived polyphenols have been found to be MORE EFFECTIVE than the drug trastuzumab and AS EFFECTIVE as the drug lapatinib against HER2+ breast cancer cells. *(80)* So go ahead and eat like a Greek! Choose cold pressed EVOO since it has a higher concentration of bio-active compounds than refined oil. *(17)*

Mushrooms

Mushrooms types including shiitake, maitake, enokidake, cremini, portobello, oyster, and thistle oyster all contain lentinan which stimulates the reproduction and activity of immune cells. *(17)* Lentinan, has been well studied and is thought responsible for the mushroom's beneficial effects. It has been shown to have anticancer effects in colon cancer cells. *(81)* Eat your 'shrooms.

Garlic/Onions/Leeks/Shallots/Chives

This group is called the allium family, and members contain sulfur compounds which have been found to cause cell death in colon, lung, breast, and prostate cancers as well as leukemia. Such sulfur compounds reduce the cancer-causing effects of nitrosamines which are created in over-grilled meats, making them helpful in cancer prevention. All the herbs in this family also play a role in regulating blood sugar levels. *(17)* Alliums family veggies also contain polyphenols, including the flavonoid quercetin, which along with many of the sulfur compounds have important anti-inflammatory effects. *(82)* It is no wonder, then, that garlic has been used for ages as a medicinal herb. Prescriptions for garlic have been found on Sumerian tablets from 3000 B.C. *(17)* From Roman times through World War I, garlic poultices were used to prevent wound infections. Louis Pasteur performed some of the original work showing that garlic could kill bacteria. Garlic was even called Russian Penicillin during World War II because, after running out of antibiotics, the Russian government used garlic poultices treatment for its soldiers. (83) Since members of this family offer many potential health benefits, don't be shy about using them to add flavor to your favorite dishes! (*Side note: though this is a group of nutritional powerhouses, this family of food actually causes an inflammatory response in some individuals. This is especially true for those who have autoimmune disorders. Pay attention when you eat these and note any adverse reactions like skin rashes, headaches, etc.)

Other Notable Foods

Countless books with specific studies of particular foods and their health benefits could be filled.....and maybe I'll do that one day. But for now, I have to move on before we run out of paper. A few foods possessing notable benefits for cancer prevention are seaweed (yes, I said seaweed), wine (thank goodness....I should mention that the daily recommended amount for benefit is one glass...and that you should look for sulfate-free wine), and dark chocolate (more than 70 percent cocoa). (17)

Grab some sushi rolled with seaweed, a side of seaweed salad, a glass of wine and some dark chocolate and let's keep pressing forward.

So far, we've talked about foods and groups of foods, but there are a few other specific nutrients that should be mentioned. They can be found in a variety of foods and all provide both general health and cancer prevention benefits.

Vitamin D

Vitamin D is a well-studied nutrient, and an important vitamin for the body. It has roles in immunity, reproduction, insulin secretion, and bone health. (70) We also know that Vitamin D3 likely protects us from colds and flu and contributes to maintaining a positive mental outlook. Vitamin D is made by your body when exposed to sunlight. This is why children living in northern latitudes are given fish cod oil (rich in Vitamin D) to prevent rickets (which results from a Vitamin D deficiency). (17) When it comes to cancer prevention, Vitamin D plays a huge role. "Strong evidence indicates that intake or synthesis of Vitamin D is associated with reduced incidence and death rates of colon, breast, prostate, and ovarian cancers." Despite more than ONE THOUSAND laboratory and epidemiological studies showing Vitamin D to reduce cancer risk, medical communities have failed to adopt the use of Vitamin D for cancer prevention. So, 1000 IU (International Units) of vitamin D3 costs less than five cents per day and there are over 1000 studies showing that it has the ability to reduce cancer incidence, and it still isn't recommended in the United states as a means for cancer prevention. Nice. "The National Academy of Sciences recommends the following daily intakes of vitamin D: 1 to 50 years of age, 200 international units (IU); 51 to 70 years, 400 IU; older than 71 years, 600 IU." (84) The best dietary sources of Vitamin D are cod liver oil (1460 IUs in a tablespoon), salmon, mackerel, and eel. Milk is usually fortified with Vitamin D, but it only contains 98 IUs per glass. (17) Vitamin D is a fat soluble vitamin, so that means excess amounts can be stored in the body. Ergo toxicity is possible. Vitamin D up to 1000 IUs per day has "no reasonable likelihood of producing toxicity". (84) If you are to take more, you should be having blood levels monitored every three months by a lab work. (17) I pour as much whole, nutritious food into my body as possible, and Vitamin D is one of the supplements I take daily.

Omega 3 Fatty Acids

We need omega-3 fatty acids for numerous normal body functions. They help control blood clotting and they help build our cell membranes in the brain. "Omega-3 fatty acids are also associated with many health benefits, including protection against heart disease and possibly stroke. New studies are identifying potential benefits for a wide range of conditions including cancer, inflammatory bowel disease, and other autoimmune diseases such as lupus and rheumatoid arthritis." Our body does not make omega-3 fatty acids, so we must get them through our food. (85)

Recall earlier in the chapter that we talked about how the typical Western diet is high in omega-6 fatty acids. Your body does need omega-6 fatty acids. The optimal ratio of omega-6 to omega-3 fatty acids is 1:1, but the Western diet ratio is around 15:1. This leads to all sorts of inflammation and hullabaloo. The best way to bring this ratio into better balance is to avoid processed foods, which are full of omega-6 fatty acids, and consume more foods rich in omega-3 fatty acids.

You may know that fatty fish such as salmon are high in omega-3 fatty acids. However, remember that the farther up the food chain you travel, the more likely that the fish is contaminated by mercury, PCBs (remember those from the endocrine disrupting chapter), and dioxin. Though such fish can be part of a healthy diet, you don't want to consume them too often because of the contaminants. Some of the best sources of fatty fish which fall lower on the food chain are small fish such as whole anchovies, small mackerel, and sardines (packed in olive oil and not sunflower oil, since sunflower oil is high in omega-6 fatty acids). However, the richest source of omega-3 fatty acids is actually a plant. In fact, 3 of the top 5 sources are plants. Listed from greatest amount of omega-3s for a 200 calorie serving, the top five sources are: flaxseed oil, flax seeds, salmon fish oil, chia seeds, and Agutuk. Other notable sources include walnuts and walnut oil, fresh basil, and grape leaves. (86) One of the easiest way I increase my intake of omega-3 fatty acids is by throwing chia or flax seeds in my smoothies.

Probiotics/Prebiotics

Probiotics and prebiotics...what's the difference? "Probiotics are good bacteria that help keep your digestive system healthy by controlling growth of harmful bacteria. Prebiotics are carbohydrates that cannot be digested by the human body." Basically prebiotics serve as food for probiotics. Prebiotics support probiotics by feeding them. (87) Probiotics and prebiotics have been well studied for their positive effect on digestive health. There is a growing body of research for their beneficial effects on supporting the immune system and preventing infection, malnutrition, intestinal inflammation, and cancer. (88)

Probiotics can be obtained through cultured dairy products (such as yogurt and kefir) and fermented foods like sauerkraut, kimchi, and kombucha. Look for products that contain the either the phrase "contains live cultures" or "contains active cultures". Probiotics can also be obtained through supplements. As for prebiotics to feed those good bacteria, the two best sources are chicory root and Jerusalem artichokes. (Jerusalem artichokes are not the green artichokes you likely think about when you hear the word artichoke. They are tubers...more like a potato.) Other good sources of prebiotics are root vegetables containing significant amounts of inulin. Examples include root vegetables like onion, jicama root, dandelion root, burdock root, leeks, and asparagus. Fibers found in many foods, including oats, barley, and apples can be fermented into substances that help to feed the beneficial bacteria in our intestines. For this reason, it is also possible to think about these foods as "prebiotic." If you look at it from this standpoint, high-fiber foods in general make good prebiotics in the sense that they remain undigested and serve as food for probiotics. (89)

Enzymes

Here I go again making you revisit your biology and chemistry lessons. An enzyme is something that speeds up a

188

chemical reaction without getting used up in the process. There are thousands of different enzymes in our bodies, and each of them performs specific jobs. Think of it like a specific key fitting a lock. You have to have the right enzymes for particular reactions. Over time, our enzyme supply decreases primarily due to processed foods and overuse of antibiotics. Without enough enzymes, many necessary chemical reactions cannot take place in our bodies. This leads to poor digestion and inadequate nutrient absorption. In turn, that leads to a myriad of health problems. Great sources of enzymes include papaya, pineapple, mango, kiwi, grapes, avocado, raw honey (the enzymes actually come from the bee's saliva), bee pollen, extra virgin olive oil, coconut oil, raw meat and dairy. (Cooking destroys most enzymes.) Enzymes can also be obtained through supplementation. *(90)*

Selenium Rich Foods

Selenium stimulates immune cells, especially NK cells. (Recall that NK cells are "natural killer cells" and they are very good at attacking both viruses and tumors.) Selenium can be found in the soil, so vegetables and cereal grains are good sources. However, intensive agriculture depletes farmland of its selenium content. This is yet another reason why buying organic matters. Organically grown veggies and cereals contain large quantities of selenium. Fish and shellfish are also good sources. *(17)*

Herbs/Spices

Herbs and spices offer a multitude of health benefits as well. Many of them, especially rosemary, thyme, oregano, basil, and mint, promote cancer cell apoptosis (death) and can reduce the spread of tumors to neighboring tissues by blocking the enzymes cancer cells need to do so. These herbs are rich in essential oils of the terpene family. Such oils owe their unique fragrances to the essential oils found in said terpene family. *(17)* You may have picked up hints of my love for essential oils throughout this book. The health benefits of essential oils are not limited to the terpene family, and the potential for therapeutic benefits of essential oils is enormous. (We'll revisit and further discuss this in the next chapter on natural health.)

Though there are many herbs and spices which play a role in good health, when it comes to cancer, the standout in the crowd is turmeric. It has been used in Ayurvedic medicine for centuries. In the last 30 years curcumin, one of turmeric's active compounds, has been well studied in a range of diseases including cancer, cardiovascular disease, and Alzheimer disease. It is even being used at M.D. Anderson in phase I and II cancer-related clinical trials. (91) A "large number of animal experiments support studies in the clinic with gynecological cancer, breast cancer, and bladder cancer, and the combination of curcumin with chemotherapy in pancreatic cancer". It is important to note that turmeric/curcumin on its own is not well absorbed by the human gut. It is best absorbed by mixing it with ginger or black pepper and a little bit of healthy oil. In fact, mixing it with black pepper increases the body's absorption of turmeric by TWO THOUSAND PERCENT. (17) You can increase your intake by making a whole bunch of curried food or consuming turmeric tea or golden milk. If curried food isn't your thing, you can make your own turmeric capsules or tincture. Turmeric is also available in supplement form.

So, what to sip with all that delicious, healthy food?

Of course, never discount good old fashioned water. Though it does not contain specific macronutrients or vitamins, having a well-hydrated body is imperative to good health. Water is also essential for flushing out toxins. I love straight up water on the rocks. I also enjoy spiking it with a few drops of my favorite essential oils for added health benefits. Other notable sipping options are listed below.

Tea

Tea varieties offer various antioxidants that are both good for your health and beneficial in cancer prevention. According to the National Cancer Institute, "Among their many biological activities, the predominant polyphenols in green tea—EGCG, EGC, ECG, and EC—and the theaflavins and thearubigins in black teas have antioxidant activity. These chemicals, especially EGCG and ECG, have substantial free radical scavenging activity and may protect cells from DNA damage…Tea polyphenols have also been shown to inhibit tumor cell proliferation and induce apoptosis in laboratory and animal studies." Catechins, another compound found in tea, have been shown to inhibit both angiogenesis (new blood supplies to feed tumors) and tumor cell invasiveness. Compounds in tea also protect against UVB radiation, help stimulate the immune system, and help detoxify the body. (92) Avoid pre-bottled teas, store-bought teas. These have far fewer antioxidants than fresh brewed tea and often contain preservatives, artificial coloring, and more. So, brew it fresh and enjoy as-is or sweeten with organic honey, agave, or stevia.

Pomegranate Juice

Pomegranate juice has been used in Persian medicine for thousands of years. It contains powerful antiinflammatory and antioxidant properties. Remember ellagic acid and all its goodness from the berry section? Pomegranate juice is loaded with it. It has been shown to slay prostate cancer, even when the cancer is aggressive. Progression of established prostate cancer has been shown to be reduced by 67% with daily consumption of pomegranate juice. Eight ounces per day is recommended for optimal health benefits. (17)

FOOD SYNERGY

We have already touched on food synergy a bit. Food synergy is the concept that certain foods, when consumed together, interact with each to make nutrients more available lending more health benefits. Recall that prebiotics and probiotics support one another. Black pepper increases the absorption of turmeric between 1000% and 2000%. When thinking about food synergy, nature has really always known best. Foods contain hundreds of biologically active compounds that have the potential to work together. Turns out variety really is the spice of life. Recent science has identified several stand-out combinations. Food synergy can apply to two foods consumed together, or it can mean certain nutrients consumed together in the same whole food. Some superstar combos include:

- TOMATOES + BROCCOLI = Each is full of phytonutrients which work harder together than alone. Studies have shown the combo of the two to be able to shrink prostate cancer.
- APPLES + THE PEEL = The phytochemicals in the flesh support the absorption of those in the peel. An apple a day…..eat the whole thing. Except maybe the seeds and stems. They probably wouldn't taste very good.
- TOMATOES (cooked with peel) + OLIVE OIL = Ninety eight percent of a tomato's flavonols are found in the peel and are best absorbed when cooked and consumed with a bit of healthy fat like olive oil.
- TEA + LEMON = Adding lemon to green tea can increase the amount of available polyphenols from about 20% to around 80%.
- LEAFY GREENS (kale, spinach, etc) +LEMON = The vitamin C in citrus fruits like lemon increase the absorption of the iron in leafy greens.
- TURMERIC + BLACK PEPPER = Black pepper increases the absorption of cancer-fighting turmeric by 1000-2000%.

- PREBIOTICS + PROBIOTICS = Prebiotics serve as food for probiotics.
- TOMATOES + AVOCADOS = The healthy fat in the avocados increases the absorption of the carotenoids in tomatoes.
- BERRIES (rich in ellagic acid) + OATMEAL = The ellagic acid in berries plays well with the antioxidants found in oatmeal. (Oats have higher antioxidant levels than most grains.)

EATING HEALTHY ON A BUDGET

When it comes to eating healthy, the two excuses I hear the most often are: "Eating healthy is too expensive" and "Eating healthy takes too much time". I beg to differ on both accounts. As with most anything, if you want it badly enough, you will find a way. If you don't, you will find an excuse. I plan to have my next book include easy, inexpensive options. If you give "eating healthy on a budget" or "organic meal for $5" a Google, you will come up with tons of ideas. The average fast food "value" meal costs between $5 and $7, but is there really anything of "value" to it? You will get processed foods foods full of chemicals, preservatives, additives, artificial colors, and calories, while the food will typically be lacking in vitamins, minerals, and phytochemicals. In fact, studies have shown that eating fast food is in fact far more expensive than preparing meals at home. The annual average for a convenience-type diet was around TWICE as much as a healthy, home-prepared diet. *(101)* Now, before you go all "but I don't have time to cook 3 meals a day at home". I get it. I agree. A meal doesn't have to be something you spend hours cooking. You have to change your perspective of how your meal looks. There are lots of tricks. A fruit or fruit & veggie smoothie takes about 3-4 minutes from start to finish including cleanup if you use frozen fruits/veggies. Toast and organic nut butter with a banana, and you are out the door in 3 minutes. Veggies, hummus, and fruit plate....super zippy. Avocado spread on Ezekial bread...

boom. Super fast. When you cook bigger meals like soups, spaghetti, etc, take advantage of your slow-cooker and let it do most of the work for you...and prepare more than you need for one sit-down meal. Freeze leftovers and you can have a homemade healthy meal in a snap. Make small changes here and there, and before you know it, you have completely overhauled the way you approach your diet.

Some general guidelines for eating healthy without robbing a bank:

- Buy whole foods. The majority of pre-packaged foods are both more expensive and less nutritious than whole foods.
- Organic is important. If you cannot buy all organic, try to avoid the Dirty Dozen. The Dirty Dozen includes foods with the highest residues of pesticides. The DD for 2018: strawberries, spinach, nectarines, apples, grapes, peaches, cherries, pears, tomatoes, celery, potatoes, sweet bell peppers.(102)
- Buy in-season fruits and veggies, because in-season is less expensive.
- Join your favorite company's social media pages for sales and coupons.
- Do-it yourself when it comes to granola bars, kale chips, smoothies, juices, soups, hummus, etc.
- Make use of your freezer. Buy in season when items are cheaper and freeze excess. Prepare food ahead and freeze. Get creative.
- Remember that you can get high quality protein from beans, quinoa, buckwheat, hemp seeds, chia seeds, sprouted-grain bread, hummus, nuts and more....and typically for far less money than meat and dairy.
- Grow your own, if that is your thing. Plant a small garden in the backyard or a container garden on your front steps or balcony.

•Don't have the best resources nearby? Go online....order in bulk.

TO SUM IT UP

Eat as close to the Earth as you can. Processed foods will do you no favors. Food is fundamental, but technology over the past 100 years or so has created so much food that is fundamentally wrong. The act of processing food hasn't even been around that long. In its short presence in the timeline of humanity, it has done much damage to our health. It began with industrialized roller milling and mass refining of grains around 1880. Worldwide epidemics of pellagra and beriberi ensued because of the loss of B vitamins during grain processing to remove the germ for longer shelf-life. The 1930s brought the discovery that nicotinic acid (aka niacin/Vitamin B6) was the specific nutrient to prevent pellagra and that thiamin (Vitamin B1) was responsible for preventing beriberi. Instead of modifying food production, grain products were simply fortified with niacin and thiamin. This was the advent of the "Wonderbread" culture of stripping foods of their natural goodness and fortifying them with synthetic supplements in the name of mass production.

Processed, mass production of foods has resulted in a loss of food synergy and an increase in chronic disease. Because foods contain hundreds of biologically active compounds, the magic is in the synergy. So, I urge you to say no to processed junk and *yes* to foods that will *nurture* you. Say *yes* to *variety*. Say *yes* to a *multitude of colors on your plate*. Say *yes* to *unadulterated foods*.

Say *yes* to your *health*.

Fifteen

Natural Health

Natural Health

When it comes to our health, often we do not pay much attention until we start to lose it. It is when faced with a life-threatening illness or when we begin to suffer daily in pain from chronic illness that attention to our health takes priority. Wholly losing my health at age 36 made me question so many things. What I discovered was that many of the answers to those questions infuriated me. I don't think I am alone. I think that many are dying for change, and sadly for some, that is a very literal statement.

I find that so many people are sick and tired of being sick and tired. Tired of getting sick and fat without even trying because of the sad state of our food supply. Over being told that the only way to cure ailments and disease is with a pill. There is neither a pill to override chronic, poor lifestyle choices nor a pill to override the exposure to harmful ingredients that companies use (while they keep us in the dark about those ingredients). I am worn out with an FDA who tells us that we cannot make claims that food can have a huge overall impact on our health while they simultaneously approve additive after additive "safe" for consumption, even though they have a long history of approving additives they later have to disapprove because they made people sick. The very fact that the FDA has been run by the former vice president of Monsanto speaks volumes. The same FDA allows claims of treatment, management, or cure of a disease to ONLY be by drugs approved by them. For me to tell you that my allergies are managed far better by changing my diet and by adding essential oils like lavender or german chamomile than they ever were by years and years of pills is a claim of illegal drug use in the eyes of the FDA. Yep, that's me....suburban-mom-yoga-enthusiast.....drug pusher....female Walter White...cooking up essential oil fixes. If you ask me, the fact that people can use their own brains to find natural ways to alleviate their ills scares the hell out of the FDA. Since drug companies cannot patent something

100% nature-derived, they cannot profit from natural remedies. Drug companies and the FDA are super cozy with one another.

While we are talking pills, let's talk about how it makes no sense to need a prescription for a second or third pill to combat the effects of pills one and two for a disease that was preventable by lifestyle choices in the first place. You see the vicious cycle here? Now, am I telling you to blindly trust someone's claims of a natural remedy? Absolutely not. Use that information as a starting place for your own reading, conversing, and researching. Am I saying that there is no place in healthcare for pharmaceuticals? Again, I am not. I am talking about tuning into our own self care...*our own health care*...so that we give ourselves the best chance for good health.

I am also so very bothered by the fact that the World Health Organization (WHO) predicts a 70% increase in cancer over the next two decades. Let that sink in. SEVENTY PERCENT more people are expected to have cancer in TWENTY YEARS. Presently, 14 million new cancer diagnoses occur per year and 8.2 million suffer cancer-related deaths. So, we are talking 70% MORE than that. If that doesn't scare the bejesus out of you, then I don't know what would. *(1)*

As much as I am incensed by all of this, I am *equally* hopeful and optimistic. There exists a body of people hungry for change, and we are growing. It is my hope that our numbers explode into an unstoppable critical mass of change. Let's stop spending insane amounts of money to mange chronic ailments and spend more on prevention. How about racing for nipping-it-in-the-bud *just as often* as we race for cures. (And boy do we need cures.) Let's stop letting those who profit from our illness manage the only accepted and insurable treatment options. Let's take charge of our own health.

In order to take charge of our own health, we must first consider our approach to healthcare. In the United States, I think we are very good at emergency medicine. There is no better place to be if you find yourself in an accident requiring immediate, skilled care. Need some stitches? Gunshot wound? Severed limb? Car accident? Basically anything that requires critical care, and you are in a great place for treatment. We are great at emergency care. We are great at treating acute health crises. But *HEALTHcare*? I am afraid we've lost our way. I think I would call our system *SICKcare*. People want a pill to manage their ills, and *most* (not all!) doctors are more than happy to prescribe. Is it that I think doctors are not smart people? Heavens no…most doctors are brilliant. They are people who finish at the tops of their classes and go on to the most challenging schools. But, they are not taught about nutrition and natural remedies at these schools. Do I think that doctors do not want to help their patients? Again, that is a definitive no. However, because of the way our 'health'care system is designed, there is no real incentive to promote true health. There *is* plenty of incentive to write a lot of prescriptions. Repeat business is desirable. Patients also play an important role in this dynamic. Most are perfectly happy habitually popping pills to manage their ailments.

In American culture, we have been conditioned to prefer pharmaceuticals over lifestyle changes or natural approaches. The only things that can be prescribed to 'treat' a disease must be approved by the FDA. We are shaped our whole lives to fear anything not approved by the FDA. But did you know that FDA approved drugs result in 711,232 "serious outcomes" per year? (Latest data 2013) Serious outcomes "include death, hospitalization, life-threatening, disability, and congenital anomaly", so we aren't talking your run-of-the-mill rash or case of diarrhea. Of those three quarters of a million "serious outcomes", 117,752 were deaths. That is over one hundred thousand people dead in a year as a result of FDA approved drugs. Both serious outcomes and deaths from FDA approved drugs increased every single year from 2004 to 2013. I am not making this up. You can check it out on the FDA's very own website. (2) Further, these numbers only reflect *reported* cases. This data is not linked to obscure drugs, either. Acetaminophen, the active ingredient in things like Tylenol, NyQuil, Theraflu, and Exedrin, leads to around 80,000 emergency room visits, 26,000 hospitalizations and 500 deaths annually. It is a liver toxin, yet we don't think twice about popping it daily.[3]

Shake your faith in the FDA a bit? Sure does jiggle mine.

It has not always been this way. Unlike today, homeopathy, naturopathy, and nutrition education once had a place in medical training. How did we move so far away from taking the natural approach as a first line of defense when it comes to sickness? The answer involves a short history lesson and one more hop down the money trail.

We are encouraged to believe that our current setup with the American Medical Association (AMA), the FDA and medical practitioners is the way it has always been, but that isn't the case. The root of the the rift between natural medicine and synthetic pharmaceutical medicine can be traced back to the turn of the last century. The story involves the wealthy Carnegie and Rockefeller families.

Let's begin around the year 1900. At that time herbalists, homeopathic practitioners, and chiropractors were in high demand. The AMA was in existence, but it was weak, unorganized, and lacking the general respect of the public. Naturalists flourished while medical doctors struggled to make a living. So, the AMA created the Council on Medical Education in 1904 with the intent to upgrade medical education. Were this intent entirely pure, it would have been a highly worthy cause. Reform for the betterment of a system is a good thing. Yet as often is true, things were not so cut and dry. The Council on Medical Education devised a plan to rank all of the medical colleges in the United States. The actual guidelines were questionable. For example, simply having the word "homeopathic" in the name of the medical school reduced its ranking. The year 1910 rolls around, and the AMA has run out of money to complete their takeover. [4] Enter the Carnegies and Rockefellers. They were approached by MP

Callwell, secretary of the Council on Medical Education, to "finish the takeover of the health industry that the AMA had started". Around this time, the Carnegies and Rockefellers joined forces to create an education fund. To finish the reform of the medical college system that had been begun by the AMA, they moved forward with a system for ranking. Abraham Flexner was nominated by his brother Simon Flexner who was on the board of directors for the Rockefeller Institute to complete the ranking. (4) Abraham Flexner was not a doctor. He was a former school teacher and an expert on educational practices. Flexner traveled the country ranking medical schools. His basis for ranking relied heavily on the German style of medical education in which physicians were trained in a laboratory first and "had a responsibility to generate new information and create progress in medical science". (5) It was the completion of his findings, The Flexner Report, that changed the whole system. Based on The Flexner Report, the AMA "made it their job to target and shut down the larger respected homeopathic colleges". At this time, both the Carnegies and the Rockefellers had begun to pour hundreds of millions of dollars into medical schools that were teaching drug-intensive medicine.

Guess who was manufacturing large amounts of chemical pharmaceuticals at the time? A gold star for you if you said the Carnegies and Rockefellers. They also began to "load up the boards of directors" of these approved medical schools with people who were literally on the payroll of the donors. So, once that was in place "the course of study in those universities swung completely in the direction of pharmaceutical drugs. And it has remained that way ever since". In order to keep the financing, such universities were required to continue teaching drug-oriented material exclusively, with no inclusion of natural medicine or nutrition. Over time, this resulted in the closing of naturopathic and homeopathic colleges. By 1950 all universities teaching homeopathy were closed. (4) The Flexner model remains in place today as the foundation for the American medical system. Though

Flexner's system set the stage for amazing advances in scientific discovery, it "created an imbalance in the art and science of medicine". Thomas Duffy sums it up nicely in his paper "The Flexner Report - 100 Years Later". In it he says "There was a maldevelopment in the structure of medical education in America in the aftermath of the Flexner Report. The profession's infatuation with the hyper-rational word of German medicine created an excellence in science that was not balanced by a comparable excellence in clinical caring. Flexner's corpus was all nerves without the lifeblood of caring". *(5)*

Doctors today are truly caught in the middle. On one side, they have the pharmaceutical industry which funnels massive amounts of money into the medical system while offering easy, band-aid like solutions. Pharmaceutical companies *want* people to *rely* on their medications rather than taking matters into their own hand and discovering ways to get to the root of their health issues and address them. They advertise in slick ways, encouraging people to keep eating crap and take their Lipitor. (*The drug Lipitor is the pharmaceutical industry's biggest money maker, bringing ing a MILLION dollars an HOUR, 365 days a year at its sales peak. That equals 9 BILLION dollars a year, y'all.) *(6)* Never mind that the side effects of Lipitor include: Most common: headache, hoarseness, lower back or side pain, pain or tenderness around the eyes and cheekbones, painful or difficult urination, stuffy or runny nose Less common: abdominal or stomach pain, back pain, belching or excessive gas, constipation, general feeling of discomfort or illness, heartburn, indigestion, stomach discomfort, loss of strength, nausea, shivering, sweating, trouble sleeping and vomiting. *(7)* But hey…people want their pills! On the other side of the squeeze, there is the food industry protecting its own interests and profits at the expense of the health of the public. Then you have doctors in the middle of these two industry giants who have one thing in common: no desire to change for that would cut into their profits.

It is pretty clear to see that change is not going to come from the top down, so the only way it *is* going to happen is from the bottom up. We really have to take the bull by the horns when it comes to our own health. It is pretty simple really. Start by paying attention to what you put on and in your body. We just spent two whole chapters talking about it. Stop showering and slathering in chemicals. Stop the monsoon of chemicals and additives in the food you eat and feed your children. Oh, and get moving. We didn't dedicate a chapter to exercise, but you know that moving does a body good. There are many options...
walk....dance....run...yoga......bike ride...Pilates....turn cartwheels...hike....jump on the trampoline....get creative. Find something you love.

In the cases of natural medicine and complementary therapies, there are numerous approaches. Most of them involve attention to all of what we just talked about: reducing your toxic load, eating well, exercising, and resting. There exists herbal medicine, acupuncture, reflexology, essential oils, yoga therapy, and more. If you are really lucky, you will find a doctor with knowledge in some of these areas and with an approach to total wellness. However, most American doctors follow the Flexner protocol we discussed earlier. David Servan-Schreiber, MD touches on this in his book "AntiCancer: A New Way of Life". He talks about the paradox of "If it were true, we'd know about it". Doctors are always looking for scientific advancements to help their patients. They subscribe to journals and attend conferences, which leads them to feel that they are aware of everything going on in their field. In essence, they *are* very well informed. They are informed of large-scale double-blind studies that have been carried out on a large number of scientists. (It should be noted that these large scale studies are typically funded by large scale pharmaceutical companies.) Smaller scale studies, even those published in wonderful publications like *Nature* or *Science* often go unnoticed since doctors simply do not have time to explore the huge body of work being carried out in labs or on a smaller scale.

So, "unless they hear about these results from their typical sources, they tend to think 'it can't be true, or I'd know about it'". Further complicating the issue is the amount of money it takes to study and bring a drug to market. For example, bringing a new cancer drug to the market costs between 500 million and a billion dollars. Wowsers. That is a ton of money, but worth it to pharmaceutical companies since bringing such a drug like Taxol (an anti-cancer medicine) to market brings in a BILLION DOLLARS A YEAR to the company who holds the patent. Since you cannot patent natural substances like herbs, healthy food, lifestyle changes, and essential oils, no pharmaceutical company stands to profit from them. (6) Therefore no one can afford to finance large-scale studies on natural substances even when they show HUGE potential for successful primary or complementary treatment. It is my hope that we will see this change in my lifetime.

Outside of a healthy diet and exercise, one of my favorite facets of natural health is essential oils. Several years ago had you asked me what an essential oil was, I would have told you it was simply something that smelled nice. I had no idea about the therapeutic benefits that can be achieved with pure, quality, unadulterated essential oils.

Essential oils are the natural aromatic compounds found in the seeds, bark, stems, roots, flowers and other parts of plants. They give plants their distinctive smells, and they provide plants with protection against predators and disease. Turns out, the compounds they produce for their own health can be beneficial for ours as well. Essential oils are fat soluble, yet they do not contain fatty acids like those found in vegetable and animal oils. Their unique, fat soluble chemical structure allows them to be immediately absorbed by the skin. This also allows pure essential oils to rapidly penetrate cell membranes, travel throughout the body, and enhance cellular function. So, essential oils are not technically 'oils', but they do work well with oils.

The vast and incredible plant kingdom continues to be the subject of a plethora of research and discovery. In fact, many prescription drugs are based on naturally occurring plant compounds. Pure, unadulterated essential oils are considered by many to be the missing link in modern medicine. They are presently represented in around 10,000 medical studies. Go to pubmed.gov and see for yourself. However, though knowledge of their healing properties seems to have been lost through the years, the use of essential oils is not new. In fact, they can be considered Man's first medicine. Records dating back to 4500 B.C. describe the use of essential oils for religious and medicinal applications. Ancient writings even suggest that primordial people had an even greater understanding of essential oils than we have today

      Though potent, essential oils rarely generate negative side effects. The secret to this seems to lie in the complexity and synergy of their chemical makeup. Somehow, they avoid disrupting the body's natural balance or homeostasis. One drop of an essential oil can have several hundred different chemical structures present. It seems that if one of them has too strong an effect, another may counteract it, thus maintaining homeostasis. (If you have forgotten from Biology, homeostasis means a state of equilibrium and balance in your body.) Synthetic chemicals, in contrast, tend to have only one action and often disrupt the body's balance. Leave it to nature to create tiny drops full of such wonderment. All of this incredibly unique chemistry can allow essential oils to have a multitude of functions. That is why a particular essential oil like lavender can be beneficial for allergies, burned skin, anxiety, and more. Ergo, lavender is often called the Swiss Army knife of oils. (8, 9)

      Even though essential oils have a rich history of healing… and even though they are represented in numerous studies….and even though people share their personal experience of achieving health and wellness with them….the FDA gets really torn up if you suggest that they may be a means of easing your ills. I encourage you to explore and expand your knowledge. There are many books on the subject. "The Essential Oils Desk Reference", "The

Healing Intelligence of Essential Oils", and "Surviving When Modern Medicine Fails" are some of my favorites.

When choosing an essential oil for therapeutic purposes, it is imperative to choose an unadulterated oil. Synthetic oils or oils with additives can cause a great deal of harm. Kurt Schnaubelt, PhD explains it very well in his book "The Healing Intelligence of Essential Oils". He points out that an absolute ocean of processed oils lie between the seeker and true, authentic, unadulterated essential oils. Further, he explains that "*Authentic* essential oils initiate processes designed by evolution arising at the level of the whole plant organism. *Adulterated* essential oils initiate processes arising at the interface of smart engineering and the corporate objective to cut cost.". So, adulteration results in a cheaper, less effective, and possibly dangerous essential oil that earns the producing company a nice profit. Schnaubelt stresses that the only way to know for a fact that an oil is genuine, authentic, uncut, and unadulterated is to know the source of the oil. The company you choose should be be able to trace the oil all the way back to its origin as a seed. They should also ensure that non-toxic extraction techniques are used.

I have personally experienced so many positive things from essential oil use for both myself and for my family. In the area of cancer in particular, there were many things I used to ease my symptoms during treatment. I continue to use other oils to restore my health. "The Healing Intelligence of Essential Oils" has an entire chapter dedicated to essential oils and cancer treatment. The chapter includes suggestions for all sorts of things to alleviate the deleterious side effects of cancer treatment. Schnaubelt references a very important body of work highlighting the great value of essential oils in cancer treatment by Dr. Anne-Marie Giraud-Robert. She is a French physician who conducted a nine year study of 1800 stage 3 and stage 4 cancer patients undergoing conventional and essential oil therapy concurrently. The study was presented in 2009, and it showed that those who received essential oil treatments along with conventional treatments had significantly higher survival rates than patients with comparative cancers who received conventional treatments alone. This was true for lung, colon, uterine, and breast cancer, as well as for all other types of cancer that were observed. Pretty amazing stuff! Since most essential oils have multiple beneficial effects, they can do everything from acting against infectious organisms to healing tissue to stimulating appetite to acting as gentle antidepressants. (9)

Just like with the subjects of exercise, eliminating toxins, and eating quality food, I could go on forever and a day about natural health and essential oils. For this book though, we are at the end of the road. It is my hope that you will use some of this information to create and foster your own wellness, purpose, and abundance. I hope you will feel that it is unacceptable to continue to be the victim of big pharma and the food industry in the name of their profits. Again, this is not a call to ditch modern medicine completely, rather it is a suggestion to seek wellness through natural measures as your first line of defense. I hope that you will make changes beginning today. It doesn't matter where you are when you start. Maybe you are already in tune to your health and you simply want to continue down the right path. Perhaps your starting place is much different. Maybe you are beginning from a broken-and-falling-apart-at-the-seams-in-every-aspect-of-your-life-from-health-to-finances place. Whatever place in the spectrum you find yourself, it really doesn't matter. The only important thing is to start. Start big or start small....just start. After all, "The Mississippi is mighty, but it starts in Minnesota, with a place that you could walk across with five steps down". All journeys big and small start in the same way....with that first step.

If you would like to keep abreast of updates, explore more health-related topics, and more, follow along through my website.

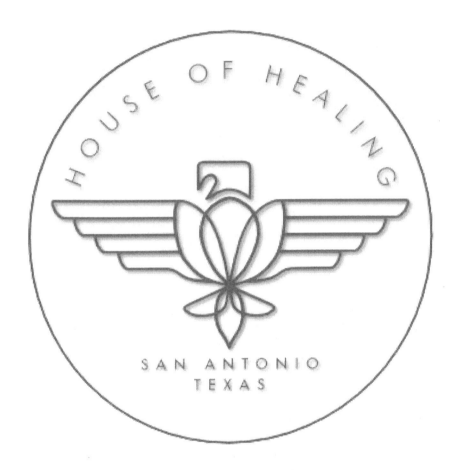

www.YourHouseOfHealing.com

Wishing you much health and a lovely, happy life!
May wellness, purpose, and abundance be yours.

XOXO,
Natalie

Appendix

Of Handy Tips

PREPPING FOR CHEMO

I know I mentioned before that for me, feeling prepared helps quell anxiety of the unknown. Find below some tips for chemo that will hopefully help reduce your burden of worry.

- *Comfortable clothes.* Chemo can last anywhere from an hour to many, many hours, so you'll want to be comfy. If you have a port, a loose neckline or a button-down help make the port more accessible. If you don't have a port, loose or short sleeves will be necessary for accessing your veins.

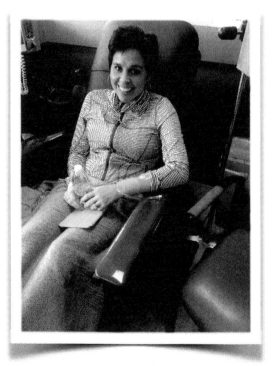

- *Cozy blanket.* Your chemo treatment room will surely have some, but there is something about having your own that makes it better. A security blanket of sorts, I guess.
- *Warm socks.* The chemo room is typically chilly. Also, if your infusion includes taxotere, you may be wearing ice glove and ice socks for an hour or more to help prevent neuropathy. You'll want a nice way to warm your tootsies afterward.

- *Water. Water. Water.* Staying well-hydrated is important. This helps prevent headaches and aids in flushing the chemo from your body. Worried about having to pee? That's ok - you just wheel your IV pole to the restroom with you.
- *Fave snacks.* Keeping something bland on my tummy helped with nausea. The chemo room will probably have snacks, but they may not be what you want. This is especially true as chemo progresses when you may have developed some food aversions. So, take something that tastes good to you.
- *Books or magazines.*
- I*pad or computer (with headphones).* Great for drowning out the hum of all the chemo room sounds. I am an avid-reader, but as chemo progressed, I found it hard to concentrate on books. Find a good series to binge watch!
- *Coloring book or puzzle.* Great for passing the time.
- *A friend or caregiver* to keep you company, to advocate for you, and to drive you home.
- *Lip conditioner.* Chemo tends to dry the lips.
- *Hard candy.* Peppermint &/or ginger are both great for combatting nausea.
- *Favorite essential oils* which can help ease your mind and aid in easing nausea. (See my blog for suggestions: www.YourHouseOfHealing.com)

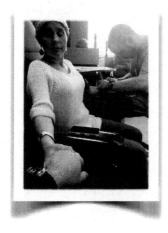
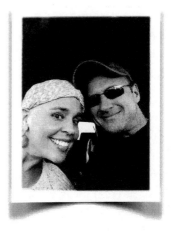

PREPPING FOR MASTECTOMY

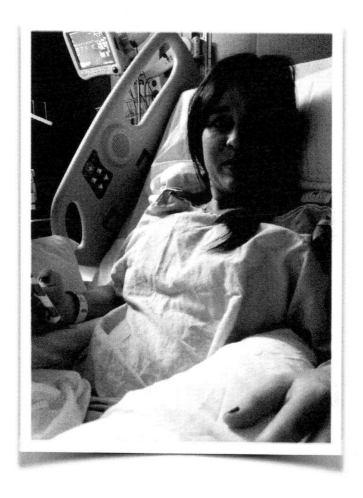

If you or someone you love is prepping for mastectomy surgery, find below some helpful tips. And if you are the one doing the prepping, you are likely feeling nervous and overwhelmed. So. Breathe in. And breathe out. Know that you are not alone. Know that you've got this.

That's me in the pic above, the morning after my bilateral mastectomy and node dissection. I was sore, tired, and nauseous. But I was determined to rise.

I hope that the following tips will help take something off your plate. I also hope that feeling well-prepared will soften some of your anxiety about the whole thing. And, sweet sister, remember the beauty of *hope*. Just as challenge can be transformed into strength, despair can be turned into hope. It is hope that can allow us to both enjoy and find peace in the present. Hope can replace worry with peace. If we look toward hope, we can allow the shadow of burden to fall behind us.

If you'd like direct links to the products listed below, head to my website: www.YourHouseOfHealing.com . You'll find this info under the blog post "Tips for Mastectomy".

ADVANCE PREP: 2-4 WEEKS PRE-OP

Soothe your soul with books, music, and meditation practices.

- "50 Days of Hope: Daily Inspiration for Your Journey through Cancer" by Lynn Eib. *I read and re-read this one.*
- Album "Soul Vibrations" by Sol Rising. *Pop in your earbuds and disappear for a bit. Relax. Meditate. Visualize healing.*
- App "Headspace". *Great for meditation.*
- Practice Yoga Nidra with me. *Check out my Instagram TV feed (@houseofhealing_) or check my website (www.YourHouseOfHealing.com) for other updates.*
- "Wildfire" magazine. This is a magazine for fighters and survivors of breast cancer. Every issue is a breath of fresh air. Plus, it is ad-free!

Speak with other survivors about the emotions that may come after mastectomy. I have a blog post about this titled "13 Scars".

Think about food for your recovery period. Prep and freeze in advance...set up a Meal Train...or both!

Clean and tidy your home. Get things the way you want them before surgery. Check out Cleaning for a Reason for your post-surgery period (or for chemo or other treatments). Cleaning for a Reason gives the gift of free house cleaning to women undergoing treatment for any type of cancer.

Shop for *drain management*. I was really unprepared for drains! Here are some things that will make the whole drain situation much easier:

- A *lanyard* for showering. The hospital will likely provide you with one. If not, there exists a nice one by Heal in Comfort. (See my website for direct link)
- I also found *shower stool* to be extremely helpful. Showering may not sound like an exhausting thing, but after a major surgery, it is. Having somewhere to sit felt safe.
- A *comfy robe* is nice. I love the company AnaOno for this. AnaOno was founded by a breast cancer survivor and offers pretty bras, robes, and loungewear.

Shop for *sleeping*.

- Soft and stretchy *button down PJs.*
- Some women prefer sleeping in a recliner, but I wanted to stay in my own bed. A good *wedge pillow* was my best friend.
- A couple of *small pillows* for under your arms. These also come in handy for car rides. You can use something you already have, but keep in mind that sometimes incisions will bleed and stain. I love *Axilla-Pillas.*
- A *sleeping mask* or an *eye-pillow* can be helpful as well. Sometimes you want to sleep in a lit hospital room, so having a

way to block out the light is nice. A sleeping mask works well. My personal favorite is a lavender eye pillow for the added benefit of a soothing aroma.

- *Essential oils* can aid in relaxation.

Shop for *post-surgery clothing.*

- *Bras and camisoles.* I love everything by AnaOno. The company was founded by a survivor for fighters and survivors. I love that pretty, feminine options for the post-surgical period and beyond are offered. AnaOno has swimwear, too! Another good option for bras is the company Wear Lively. Though not designed specifically for post breast-surgery, they offer lots of soft, wire-free bras that I have found to be comfy post surgery. (This option would be for down the road a bit…after incisions have healed and drains have been removed.)
- *Bottoms.* Remember that it will be difficult to bend over for a while, so pants can be tricky. Avoiding buttons, zippers, and tight-fitting bottoms is ideal. Elastic waist things - joggers, knit skirts and pants) make this easier. I found it useful to sit on the edge of the bed when getting dressed.
- *Tops.* Loose fitting, button down shirts work well. Lightweight, loose comfy knit tops and comfy sweaters are great, too. I recommend something with large armholes and a large neck opening if it isn't button down.

Shop for *hospital stay.* (See also everything listed above. Things listed below haven't been mentioned yet.)

- *Lip conditioner.* Lips get soooooo dry in the hospital.
- Cozy, non-skid *socks.*
- *Face wipes,* so you can freshen up right in your bed.
- Large *insulated cup,* because hospital cups are often small and they sweat. I prefer stainless steel.

- Also don't forget: comfortable underwear, a hairbrush or hat for warmth depending on the status of your noggin at the time of surgery, slip on shoes, toothbrush, books or magazines, music.

Shop for travel.

- *The Breast and Chest Buddy Seatbelt Cover* makes car-rides more comfortable as you heal.
- *Axilla-Pillas* are great under your arms while you are a passenger as they absorb bumps in the road. (Remember these are great for sleeping as well.)

HERE WE GO: 1-2 DAYS PRE-OP

- Pack your hospital bag. Use the above suggestions as a guideline.
- Remind your caregiver to pack his or her bag. Helpful items: a blanket from home, cash for vending machines, a notebook for recording details from doctors, prescription medications, as change or two of clothing, phone/computer chargers.
- A game plan for your caregiver to provide updates to family and friends.
- Exercise....meditate...get a message...pray. Do anything that will help you mentally, physically, and spiritually prepare your body for surgery.
- Have a good laugh! Tap into anything that cracks you up - whether it is a funny friend, a funny caregiver, a funny movie, or just your own sense of humor. Remember, laughter softens life's hardest blows!

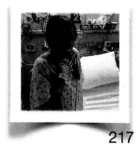

RECOVERY TIPS

- Rest. Rest. And rest some more. Your body has just been through incredible trauma. You need down time to restore. To regenerate. To heal. I love yoga nidra (guided meditation) as a deeply healing practice. (Check my Instagram @houseofhealing_ for links to practice right in the hospital or at home.)
- Balance your rest with gentle movement. Using your arms will aid in healing and help restore range of motion. You will have weight restrictions (per your doctor's recommendations) for a while, and you will likely need to avoid lifting your arms overhead until your drains are removed. In the beginning, just use your arms for daily tasks like brushing your teeth, eating, etc. Then you can add exercises to increase range of motion and decrease swelling. Lucky for you, that's just a few pages away.... ;-)
- Watch those drains! Avoid pinning them high on your clothing since gravity helps fluid flow. Make sure the tubes are secured, especially if they are long. If they are dangling about, they may get hung on something. (Remember I learned this the hard way hahahahaha!)
- Allow others to help you. When people offer to help, take them up on it! People genuinely want to help, but they don't always know what to do. So, when they ask, "How can I help?", don't be afraid to speak up. It will make them happy to care for you.
- Listen to your body and its infinite wisdom. Pace yourself. Healing takes time, and it usually isn't linear. Sometimes you will feel like you are taking one step up and two steps back. Just keep stepping, sister. Progress is progress. You'll get there. Celebrate your body's strength while honoring its temporary limitations.

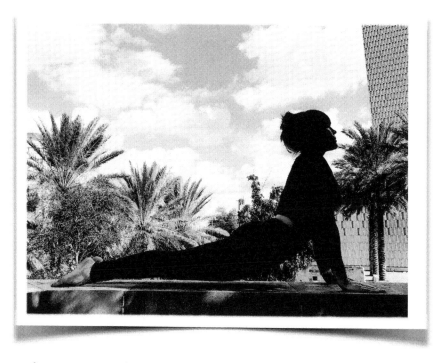

"She will rise. With a spine of steel and a roar like thunder, she will rise."
- Nicole Lyons

PINK RIBBON RESTORATION

In the pages that follow, you will find exercises that are designed to restore range of motion, to increase flexibility and stamina, to decrease swelling, and to help you reconnect with your body after breast surgery.

Always consult with your doctor before beginning any exercise program. Begin with Level 1, and progress to Level 2 only after you've been able to work through all of the Level 1 exercises. Everyone heals at different rates, so listen to your body. Take all the time you need. It isn't about how fast you get there, but as long as it takes. No need to rush. Once you've mastered Level 2, move on to Level 3 and then Level 4.

LEVEL 1

(Exercises 1-6 can be done sitting on the edge of a chair or seated in a comfortable criss-cross position on the floor.)

1. **Breathe in. Breathe out.**

Breath of Life - Left hand to heart; right hand to belly. Breathe deeply. Slowly and rhythmically. Set an intention here. Return to this intention every time you practice. (Examples: "I heal because I am alive." "My body is in a constant state of healing and regeneration." "I am restoring strength and range of motion." "I forgive my body." Your intention can be anything on which you'd like to place your focus.)

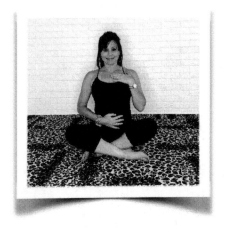

Umbrella Rib Breath
Rest your hands on the lower part of your rib cage. With each inhale, feel the ribcage expand to its full capacity, from the front of the chest all the way to the spine. Imagine an umbrella opening. Repeat 10X.

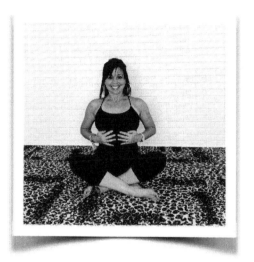

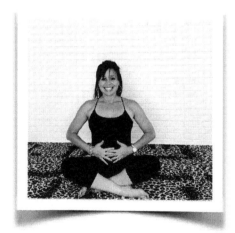

Belly Breath Place your hands on your belly so that you can feel its rise and fall. With each inhale, allow the belly to balloon and fill all the way to the pelvic floor. With each exhale, draw the pelvic floor up and the navel in. Repeat 10X

2. Neck Release

Ear to shoulder. Root down through the sit bones and grow tall through the spine, crown of the head reaching toward the ceiling. Align knees with hips and ankles with knees (if seated in a chair). Center shoulders over hips and ears over shoulders. (Repeat this start position for exercises 3-6.) Drop the left ear toward the left shoulder until you feel a nice stretch. Breathe here for several breaths, then extend the right arm to your side and slowly rotate through the shoulder joint as if you were turning a giant door knob. Repeat 5-10X then repeat on the opposite side.

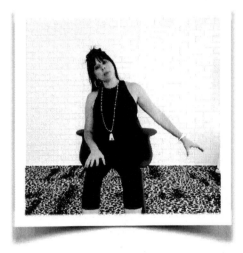

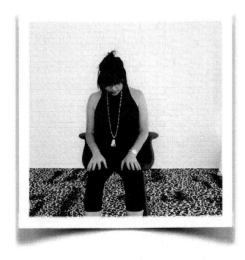

Chin to Chest With head aligned in the center, inhale deeply then drop the chin toward the chest on the exhale. Hold here for 5-10 breaths. Then with the head still dropped, gently slide your chin toward your left shoulder on the inhale - back to center on the exhale - to the right on the next inhale. Try for 5X on each side.

3. **Shoulder Rolls** Inhale and elevate the shoulders rolling them up and to the front then exhale down and back. Allow the shoulder blades to lift on the inhale then really draw them down your back on the exhale. Repeat 5-10 times in this direction then reverse the direction - inhaling with every lift and exhaling with each lower.

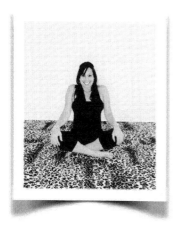 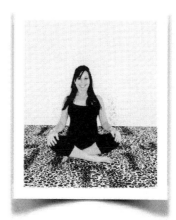

4. **Shoulder Slides** Gently scoop the belly to stabilize the core. Without arching your back, inhale to draw the shoulder blades closer together sliding the arms back. Exhale, slide the arms forward by returning the shoulder blades to their start position. Inhale and slide your arms forward feeling the space created between your shoulder blades. Repeat 5X in each direction. Be sure to keep your shoulders low and away from your ears.

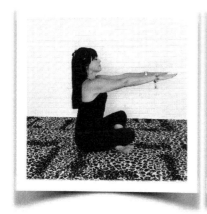 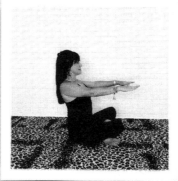

5. **Peekaboo** Keeping the shoulders low, extend your arms straight out in front of your shoulders. Spin your palms up to face the ceiling then bend your elbows 90 degrees. Keeping the elbows bent and the ribcage still, inhale and open the arms as wide as possible. Exhale, return to start. Repeat 5-10X.

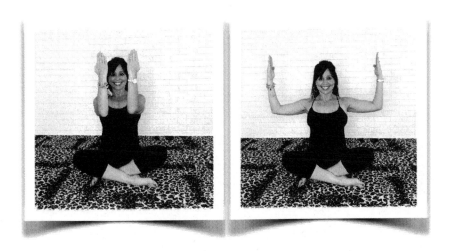

Puppet From peekaboo, keep the elbows bent, arms wide, and shoulders low. Spin your palms to face away from you. Take a deep breath in and on the exhale, rotate your right arm down while the left remains stable and still. Inhale, return to start; exhale rotate your left arm down. Continue for 5 rounds.

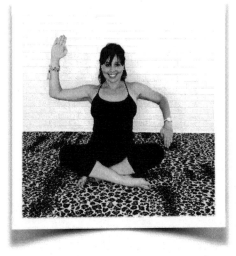

6. **Seated Cat / Cow** Inhale, lifting chin and chest and arching the back as much as is comfortable. Exhale, round forward drawing the belly in while casting your gaze toward your belly. No need to rush here - move slowly with the rhythm of your breath. Inhale - lift, expand, receive. Exhale - round and release.

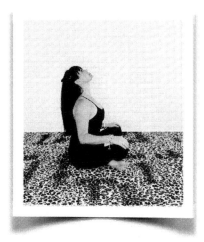 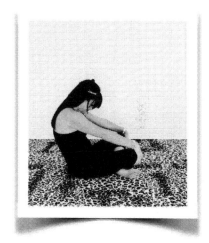

7. **Pendulum Arm** Standing with feet a bit wider than hip distance and knees slightly bent, lean forward stabilizing your left arm on your left thigh and allow your right arm to hang loosely. Let it dangle. Then make small circles allowing momentum to move the arm around effortlessly in a clockwise circle for 10 revolutions. Then reverse to counter-clockwise for 10 revolutions. Then repeat with your left arm.

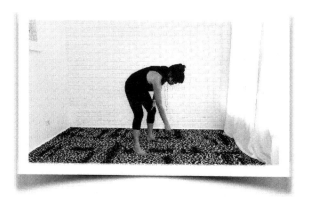

LEVEL 2

8. **Lotus to Prayer** Begin in a comfortable seated position. Bend your elbows and bring your palms together at heart center. Keeping your thumbs and pinkies together, part your middle fingers so that your hands resemble a lotus flower. Close your eyes and breathe here remembering that you have the ability to rise from the mud, bloom out of the darkness, and radiate into the world.

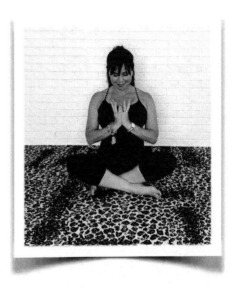

At your own pace, inhale and reach your arms wide and overhead; exhale and bring your palms together. Inhale and hold; exhale and bring your palms to heart center. Pressing your palms together and keeping your shoulder blades low, continue breathing here for 2 or 3 breath cycles. Then inhale, reach your arms wide and overhead again and repeat the whole process 2-3 times. Take time while breathing to set an intention for your practice.

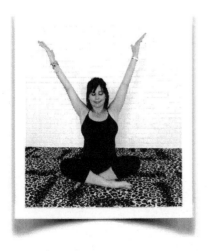

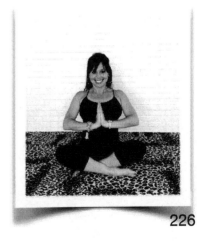

9. **Overhead Lift** Seated or standing, spine long and tall. Arms slightly in front and slightly wider than shoulder width. Inhale and gently pull the stretch band until you feel resistance. Keeping your shoulders low, lift your arms overhead with an exhale. Inhale, lower arms to start position. Repeat 5-10X, continuously drawing your shoulder blades down your back.

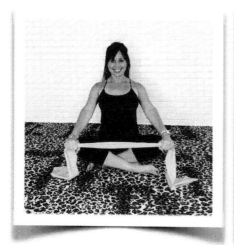 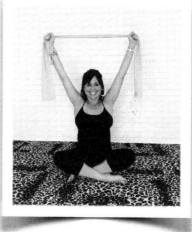

10. **Rotation** Begin in a comfortable seated position on the edge of a chair or on the mat. Arms bent with elbows wide, fingertips on your shoulders (or on top of your head if your range of motion doesn't allow for shoulders yet). Root down through your sit bones; inhale to grow tall. Exhale drawing your navel closer to your spine and twist your upper body to the right; inhale back to the center. Exhale and twist to the left, inhale and return to center. Keep your sit bones rooted, your hips square, and your belly engaged throughout. Repeat 3-4 times on each side.

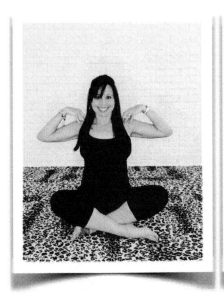 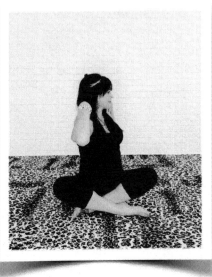

11. **Flexion** Begin in a comfortable seated position on the edge of a chair or on the mat. Arms bent with elbows wide, hands on your shoulders (or on top of your head if your range of motion doesn't allow for shoulders yet). Root down through your sit bones; inhale to grow tall. Exhale and side bend toward the right keeping your sit bones rooted. Inhale, return to center; exhale and side bend toward the left. Repeat 3-4X on each side.

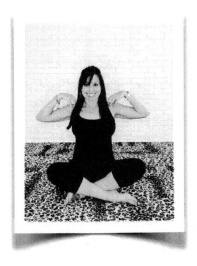 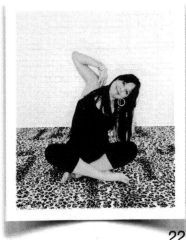

12. **Snow Angel** Lying on your back with your knees bent and your feet on the floor, begin with your arms close to your sides with palms facing down. Begin to make a snow angel by sliding the arms up. If your range of motion allows you to reach shoulder-height, pause there and spin your palms to face the ceiling. Continue lifting the arms until you reach the point in your range of motion where you feel slight resistance. Pause there and hold for three breaths. Then return your arms to the starting position, flipping the palms to face the floor as the arms reach shoulder height. Repeat 5-10X (Once you have reached the full range of motion and you feel stable in this exercise, you can attempt the advanced version lying on the foam roller.)

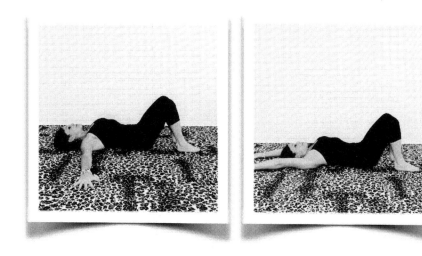

13. **Arm Scissors** Lying on your back with your knees bent and your feet on the floor, extend your arms straight toward the ceiling (perpendicular to the ground). Inhale deeply, exhale and reach the left arm overhead while the right arm reaches toward your feet. Inhale, return to start position. Exhale and repeat reaching your right arm overhead and your left toward your feet. Inhale arms back to the start position. Repeat 4 more rounds. (Once you have

reached the full range of motion and you feel stable in this exercise, you can attempt the advanced version laying on the foam roller.)

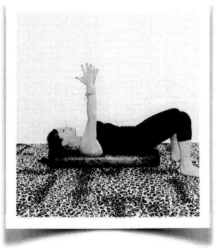 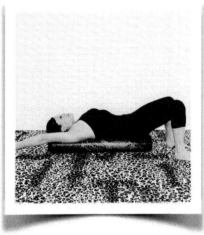

14. **Climb a Wall** (Avoid if you still have drains!) - Stand facing the wall, about arm's distance away. With your arms about shoulder-width apart, place your fingertips on the wall and begin walking them up the wall. Step forward as needed. Keep walking your arms upward until you feel tolerable resistance. Hold for eight breaths then step back and begin again, repeating 2-3X.

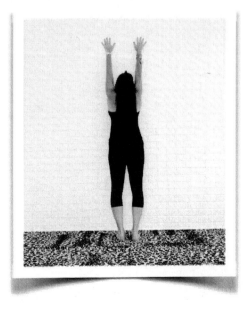

Open Pectoral Stretch (Avoid if you still have drains!) - Still facing the wall and now only a few inches away, extend your right arm straight out from your shoulder joint (parallel with the floor) and place it on the wall. Then begin to rotate your body toward the right. Keep moving your body away from the wall until you feel a nice stretch across your chest and through your right shoulder. You can soften your neck to rest your head against the wall. Hold for 8 breaths then repeat on the left side.

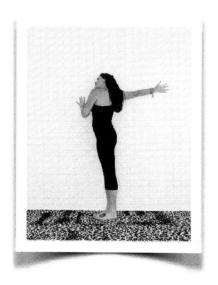

LEVEL 3

15. **Belly Fascia Breath** Begin lying on your back; knees bent; feet on the floor about hip distance apart. Place your hands on your thighs near the hip crease. Inhale deeply to draw breath all the way to your pelvic floor, allowing the belly to balloon. Exhale entirely and hold. As you hold, draw your belly button in as

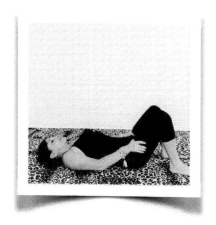

deeply as you can. At the same time, press your hands into your thighs while lifting your ribcage in the opposite direction. Hold as long as you can until you feel the need to release and inhale. Inhale deeply and repeat this process 5-10 times. As you breathe here, set an intention for your practice.

16. **Toe Taps / Psoas Stretch** Lie on your back with knees bent in tabletop position. (Advanced version can be performed laying on a foam roller.) Slide your shoulder blades down your back and draw your navel closer to your spine. Inhale to prepare; exhale tap the right toe to the mat (without changing the angle of the knee and while keeping the naval drawn in.) Inhale back to tabletop; exhale tap the left toe on the mat. Repeat 5-10X on each side.

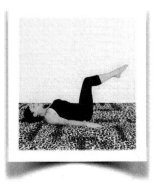 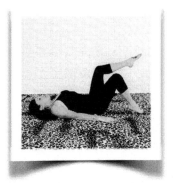

Psoas Stretch - once you are stable and confident with toe taps, you can add this exercise. Begin in table top. Inhale to prepare; exhale tap the right toe on the mat then flex the foot and extend the leg straight. Hold this stretch for three breaths, then inhale, point the toe and float your leg toward the ceiling; exhale back to table top. Do 4-8 on the right side, then repeat with the same number on the left side.

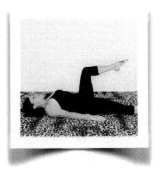 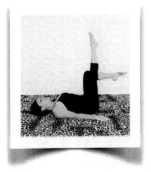

17. **Bridge** Lie on your back with your knees bent and your feet flat on the floor, approximately hip distance apart. Your feet should be in a comfortable position — neither too far from nor too close to your booty. Inhale and place a small arch in your lower back. Exhale and draw your navel in and begin to peel away from the mat lifting hips first. Inhale - hold the bridge position. Exhale, roll down slowly, one vertebrae at a time. Repeat 4 more times.

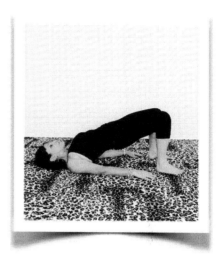

18. **Spinal Twist** Lie on your back with your knees bent and your feet flat on the floor, approximately hip distance apart. Inhale deeply, then use control to drop the knees to the right on your exhale. Keep your shoulders heavy and connected with the mat. You may rest here simply breathing or add to this by extending your left arm straight out from from your left shoulder, allowing your gaze to follow (again, you can rest here breathing deeply or continue to add by) grasping your left big toe with

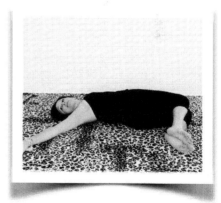

your "peace" fingers on your right hand and straightening your left leg.

19. **Neck Massage** Lie on your back with the foam roller under your neck and situated at the base of your skull. Place your hands on the ends of the roller to stabilize it. Inhale and turn your head to the right - extending it fully; exhale back to center. Inhale, rotate your head to the left; exhale back to center. Repeat for a total of 8-10 times per side.

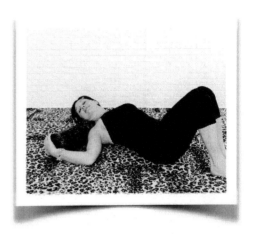

20. **Collarbone Alignment** Lie on your back with your knees bent and your feet flat on the floor; feet, knees, and inner thighs together. Place the foam roller behind your upper back on your shoulder blades, arms behind the roller on the floor with your elbows bent; palms up. Inhale deeply, then exhale and drop your knees (with control) to the right as you simultaneously look toward the left. Inhale, return to center; exhale drop your knees to the left and gaze toward the right. Repeat for a total of 8-10 times on each side. Move slowly with control.

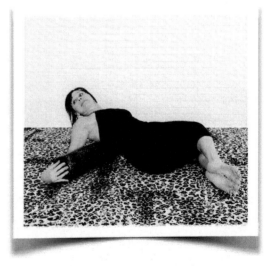

21. **Child's Pose** Kneel on the floor. Touch your big toes together and sit on your heels, then separate your knees about as wide as your hips. Exhale and lay your torso down between your thighs. Lengthen your tailbone away from the back of the pelvis while you lift the base of your skull away from the back of your neck. Lay your hands on the floor alongside your torso, palms up, and release the fronts of your shoulders toward the floor. Feel how the weight of the front shoulders pulls the shoulder blades wide across your back. Now, soften your gaze. Perhaps close your eyes.

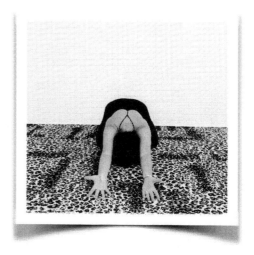

Breathe. Just breathe. And be. Just be.

LEVEL 4

Before beginning, complete a breathing exercise of your choice from Level 1, 2, or 3. (Or work through all of them!) Set an intention for your practice.

22. **Spinal Articulation** (Foam Roller) — Lie on your back with your knees bent and your feet flat on the floor about hip distance apart. Place the foam roller behind your upper back on your shoulder blades with your elbows bent and hands behind your head

235

with your fingers interlaced. Slide your shoulder blades down your back and feel an openness across your collarbones. Inhale as your arch your upper back over the roller; exhale, draw your navel inward and curl back up with control. Repeat 8-10 times.

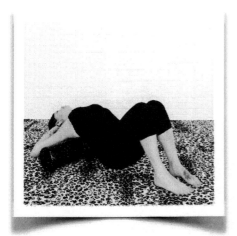 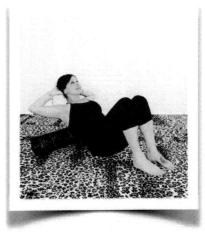

23. **Rolling Swan** (Foam Roller) - Lie on your belly. Legs are long and reaching away from your hips; arms are long and in front of you with the foam roller just below your elbows; thumbs are facing up. Draw your belly in (as if trying to lift it away from the mat). Inhale and roll the roller toward you while lifting your upper body. Arms are heavy and pressing downward, and remember to keep your belly engaged and your booty relaxed to protect your lower back. Exhale as you slowly lower down; keeping resistance on the roller. Repeat 8-10 times.

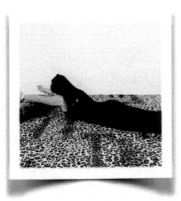 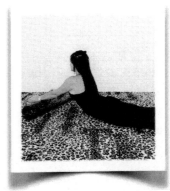

24. **Lat Pull & High Row** (Stretch Band) - Stand with the middle of the stretch band secured under your right foot, with the ends of the band in each hand. Inhale and grow tall in the spine; exhale draw your shoulder blades down and away from your ears while gently scooping your belly. Inhale again to stabilize the shoulders; exhale and press the arms straight back while keeping them straight. Repeat 6-8 times. Repeat with the same number with the band under the left foot.

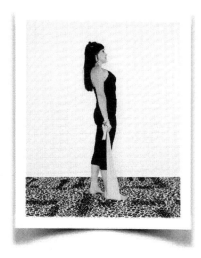
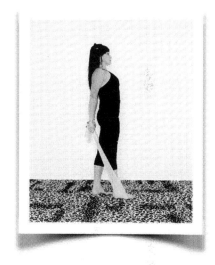

Place the band under both feet. Inhale to prepare (draw the shoulders low while gently scooping the belly); exhale, bend the elbows to pull the band upward. Keep your hands close to your body and your elbows wide and away from the body. As your elbows lift, your shoulder blades will draw closer together. Inhale to return to start, then repeat 6-8 times.

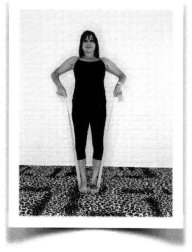

25. **Shoulder Lift Front & Side** (band) - Standing with feet shoulder width apart, place one end of the thereaband under your right foot and the other end in your right hand. (You can adjust the intensity by making the band longer or shorter.) Inhale and grow tall with a scooped belly to prepare; exhale and slowly raise your right arm up and away from the body until just below shoulder height. Be sure to keep your shoulder stable and low as your arm moves. Inhale, return to the start position; exhale and repeat 5-10 times. Repeat with the same number with the band under the left foot and with the left arm.

Repeat this exercise on both the right and left side, except this time, take your arm up and forward.

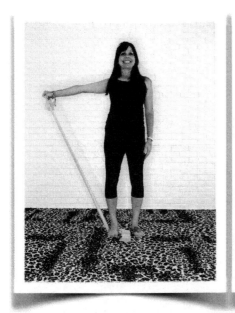 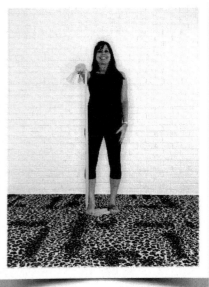

26. **Side Stretch and Pull** (band) - This exercise can be done standing or sitting.
Either way, grow long and tall in the spine and engage the core by scooping the belly. (This helps with stabilization.) Hold the theraband with the left and right hands just a bit wider than shoulder distance apart. Inhale and take both arms overhead. Exhale, bend your torso slightly to the right; stabilize the left arm (keeping it still) and pull down with the right arm. Inhale, release the right arm back to the start

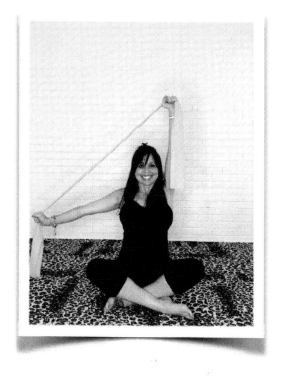

position and return your body to the upright position. Repeat 4-5 times then switch to the left side.

27. **Tadasana / Forward Fold** - Stand with the bases of your big toes touching, heels slightly apart (so that your second toes are parallel). Gently shift your weight back and forth so that it is balanced evenly on the feet. Imagine a line of energy all the way up along your inner thighs through the core of your torso, neck, and head, and out through the crown of your head. Lengthen your tailbone toward the floor Press your shoulder blades into your back, then widen them across and release them down your back. Without pushing your lower front ribs forward, lift the top of your sternum straight toward the ceiling. Widen your collarbones. Hang

your arms beside the torso, palms open and facing forward. Soften your gaze, and breathe here for about a minute.

Inhale to sweep the arms overhead bringing palms together. Exhale begin to hinge at the hips while the palms part and arms spread wide. There is a micro-bend in your knees. Continue to fold until you reach the edge of your range of motion. Breathe here for 5 breaths.

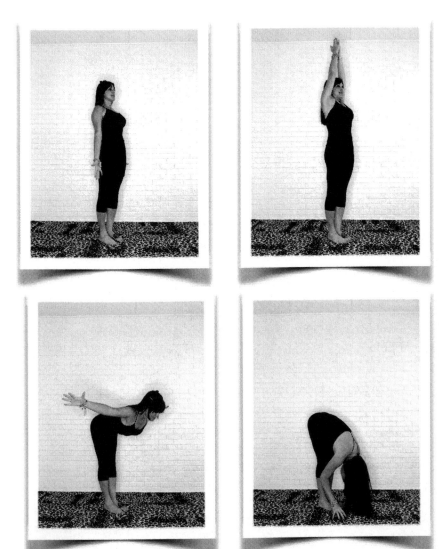

28. **Flat Back Lengthen** On your next inhale, lift until your torso is extending from your hips while being parallel to the ground. As you breathe here, focus on lifting your belly button to your spine while lengthening - crown of your head reaching away from your sit bones.

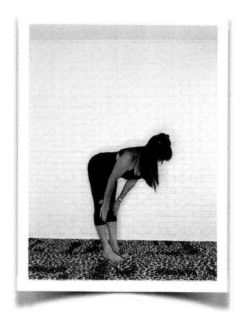

29. **Chaturanga** Exhale and bring your palms to the mat. Step or float your feet back to plank pose. Simultaneously push back through the heels to engage the quadriceps and bring the lower body to life, and reach your sternum forward, creating a straight, strong line of energy from the crown of your head through your feet. Inhale to prepare, exhale to bend your elbows to lower your body down. Keep your elbows close to your sides. Continue to lower until your shoulders are at the same height as your elbows. ***If you experience too much strain as you begin lower your body, modify by dropping to your knees first. ***

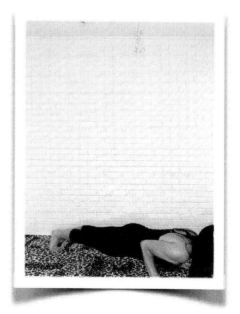

30. **Upward Dog / Downward Dog** From chaturanga, press the tops of your feet into the mat as you inhale to lift your torso up by straightening your arms. Legs remain long and strong to keep your thighs lifted off the ground while your shoulders slide away from your ears. ***If this is too much for your arms or too great a stretch for your torso, modify by keeping the legs on the ground while lifting your torso. ***

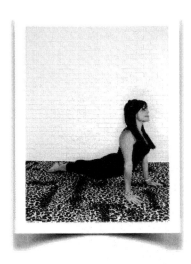 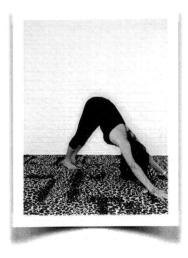

31. **Mermaid** From downward dog, lower your knees to the ground then rise to a seated position. Drop your knees to the right and swing your feet to the left. With your left hand, reach for your left ankle or left foot. Inhale and sweep your right arm overhead keeping the arm aligned with your ear; exhale and reach to the side until you feel a nice stretch in the right side body. Hold for a deep inhale, then exhale to return your arm back to the start position. Repeat 3-4 times then switch your leg position to the opposite side.

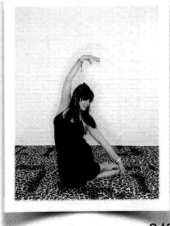

Healing You

The first two years after my cancer diagnosis were filled with treatments. One hurdle after the next. Operation after operation. Chemotherapy. Hormone therapy. Infections. An arsenal of antibiotics and anti-fungals.

When active treatment ended, I was so relieved. I was so grateful to be alive. I was so ready to get back to normal. What I didn't realize was that "normal" would forever look a little different - and - that getting to that normal would not be so straightforward.

I was released from active treatment, but I felt like a stranger in my own body. All of that poking and prodding…all of those missing body parts…all of that exposure to multiple medical personnel. I disconnected from my body in an effort to manage both physical and emotional pain. For the first time in my life, I consistently had trouble sleeping as anxieties constantly welled to the surface. My digestive system was pretty wrecked from all of that chemo and all of those meds. As joyful and full of gratitude as I was to be alive, there was an underlying dullness to me. I just didn't feel like myself. I had restored things like strength and range of motion (which felt awesome!), but I still needed restoring in other ways.

So, bit by bit, I kept researching. I kept exploring. I kept trying new things. It took a few years, but I can say that I now feel that my vitality has been restored. My current normal looks a bit different than it did before cancer, and I am ok with that because I feel happy. I feel healthy. I feel whole.

Cancer is traumatic. It turns your world upside down. You finish treatment, then you are sent on your way with little information about how to piece yourself back together. There is a gap in the space between treatment and restoration of vitality that needs to be filled. So, I have developed a program to address that gap: Healing You.

Cancer treatments can often leave the body changed, the mind foggy, and the spirit dulled. Healing You is a protocol designed to restore vitality to all three. Obtaining true well being involves working with the body as a whole - inside and out. Healing You addresses this by using rhythm, rest, nutrition education, and self-care techniques to create vibrancy.

Rhythm creates resilience in the body. Yoga and Pilates movement patterns are used to increase circulation and lymph flow throughout the body. These functional patterns optimize neuromuscular pathways to decrease inflammation and discomfort in the body while increasing mobility. Special attention is given to fascia tissue. Techniques are used hydrate and smooth out scar tissue leading to healthier, less inflamed tissues.

Rest creates resilience in the mind. It is imperative for restoration and healing. Yoga nidra, guided meditation, and breath work are all used to quiet the mind and down-regulate the nervous system. These mindful meditation techniques have been found to significantly reduce pain in experimental and clinical settings.

Chemotherapy causes profound disruption of the intestinal microbiome in terms of both composition and metabolic capacity. Dense-dose antibiotics add to this disruption. Gut health must be restored to obtain optimal wellness. Healing You addresses **nutrition education** by exploring foods which promote healing, food synergy, dense nutrition, and probiotics for the restoration of gut health.

Stress reduction, resilience mindset, toxic load reduction, and ayurvedic techniques are all utilized to create healthy habits. These practices strengthen intuitive **self care**. This conscious tending of personal well-being creates sustainable wellness.

Healing you is ultimately a wellness program for awakening healing in the body, the mind, and the spirit. I am so excited to help you build a better life after cancer, because the impact of cancer does not stop after treatment ends.

Breathe in. Breathe out. Let the healing begin!

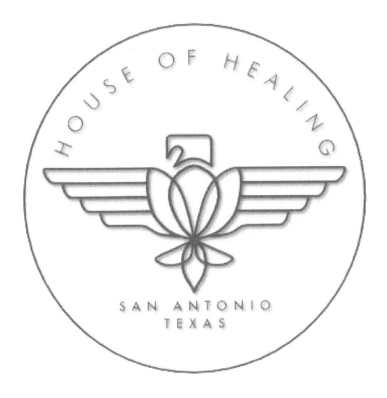

For more information about Healing You, visit my website
www.YourHouseOfHealing.com
Instagram:
@houseofhealing_

References

ENDOCRINE DISRUPTORS

1. "National Institute of Environmental Health Sciences." *Endocrine Disruptors*. N.p., n.d. Web. 22 Jan. 2015.
2. Reuben, Suzanne H. Introduction. Reducing Environmental Cancer Risk: What We Can Do Now: President's Cancer Panel 2008-2009 Annual Report. Bethesda, MD: President's Cancer Panel, 2010. N. pag. Print.
3. "Why This Matters – Cosmetics and Your Health | Skin Deep® Cosmetics Database | Environmental Working Group." *Skin Deep Why This Matters Cosmetics and Your Health Comments*. N.p., n.d. Web. 25 Jan. 2015.
4. "Body Burden: The Pollution in Newborns." Environmental Working Group. N.p., n.d. Web. 25 Jan. 2015. Environmental Working Group analysis of tests of 10 umbilical cord blood samples conducted by AXYS Analytical Services (Sydney, BC) and Flett Research Ltd. (Winnipeg, MB)
5. "National Institute of Environmental Health Sciences." Endocrine Disruptors. N.p., n.d. Web. 25 Jan. 2015.
6. Bergman, Åke, Jerrold J. Heindel, Susan Jobling, Karen A. Kidd, and R. Thomas. Zoeller. State of the Science of Endocrine Disrupting Chemicals - 2012: An Assessment of the State of the Science of Endocrine Disruptors Prepared by a Group of Experts for the United Nations Environment Programme (UNEP) and WHO. Geneva, Switzerland: United National Environment Programme, 2013. Print.
7. "Endocrine Disruptors." (n.d.): n. pag. National Institute of Environmental Health Sciences. National Institutes of Health, 01 May 2010. Web. 25 Jan. 2014.
8. Kuo, Chang-Hung, San-Nan Yang, Po-Lin Kuo, and Chih-Hsing Hung. "Immunomodulatory Effects of Environmental

Endocrine Disrupting Chemicals." The Kaohsiung Journal of Medical Sciences 28.7 (2012): S37-42. Web.

9. "Dioxins and Their Effects on Human Health." WHO. N.p., n.d. Web. 23 Jan. 2015.

10. Fraser, AJ, TF Webster, and MD McClean. "Red Meat and Poultry: Two Major Sources of PBDE Exposure in the US." — Environmental Health News. Environmental Health Perspective, 22 July 2009. Web. 26 Jan. 2015.

11. "Soft Drinks and Sports Drinks: Would You Drink Flame Retardant?" Wellness and Equality. N.p., 06 Jan. 2012. Web. 26 Jan. 2015.

12. "Pesticides." TDEX. TDEX-The Endocrine Disruption Exchange, n.d. Web. 26 Jan. 2015. <http://endocrinedisruption.org/pesticides/introduction>.

13. Colborn, Theo, and Lynn E. Carroll. "Pesticides, Sexual Development, Reproduction, and Fertility: Current Perspective and Future Direction." Human and Ecological Risk Assessment: An International Journal 13.5 (2007): 1078-110. TDEX. Web. 26 Jan. 2015. Cherednichenko, G., R. Zhang, R. A. Bannister, V. Timofeyev, N. Li, E. B. Fritsch, W. Feng, G. C. Barrientos, N. H. Schebb, B. D. Hammock, K. G. Beam, N. Chiamvimonvat, and I. N. Pessah. "Triclosan Impairs Excitation-contraction Coupling and Ca2 Dynamics in Striated Muscle." Proceedings of the National Academy of Sciences 109.35 (2012): 14158-4163. Web.<http://endocrinedisruption.org/assets/media/documents/H20850Colborn2007.pdf>.

14. Fernández-Sanjuan, María, Johan Meyer, Joana Damásio, Melissa Faria, Carlos Barata, and Silvia Lacorte. "Screening of Perfluorinated Chemicals (PFCs) in Various Aquatic Organisms." Analytical and Bioanalytical Chemistry 398.3 (2010): 1447-456. National Institute of Environmental Health Sciences. National Institutes of Health. Web. 26 Jan. 2015. <http://www.niehs.nih.gov/health/materials/perflourinated_chemicals_508.pdf>.

15. "Perfluorinated Compounds (PFCs)." Washington Toxics Coalition. N.p., n.d. Web. 26 Jan. 2015. <http://watoxics.org/chemicals-of-concern/perfluorinated-compounds-pfcs>.

16. "Pollution In People." Phthalates. Pollution in People, n.d. Web. 26 Jan. 2015. <http://pollutioninpeople.org/toxics/phthalates>.

17. Koch, Holger M., Matthew Lorber, Krista L.y. Christensen, Claudia Pälmke, Stephan Koslitz, and Thomas Brüning. "Identifying Sources of Phthalate Exposure with Human Biomonitoring: Results of a 48h Fasting Study with Urine Collection and Personal Activity Patterns." International Journal of Hygiene and Environmental Health 216.6 (2013): 672-81. Web.

18. Watkins, DJ, M. Eliot, S. Sathyanarayana, AM Calafat, K. Yolton, BP Lanphear, and JM Braun. "Variability and Predictors of Urinary Concentrations of Phthalate Metabolites during Early Childhood." Environmental Science and Technology (2014): n. pag. Web.

19. Krause M1, Klit A, Blomberg Jensen M, Søeborg T, Frederiksen H, Schlumpf M, Lichtensteiger W, Skakkebaek NE, Drzewiecki KT. Int J Androl. 2012 Jun;35(3):424-36. doi: 10.1111/j.1365-2605.2012.01280.x. Sunscreens: are they beneficial for health? An overview of endocrine disrupting properties of UV-filters.

20. "Parabens." Parabens. Breast Cancer Fund, n.d. Web. 26 Jan. 2015. <http://www.breastcancerfund.org/clear-science/radiation-chemicals-and-breast-cancer/parabens.html>.

21. Darbre PD, Aljarrah A, Miller WR, Coldham NG, Sauer MJ, Pope GS (2004). Concentrations of parabens in human breast tumors. Journal of Applied Toxicology 24:5-13.

22. Barr, L., Metaxas, G., Harbach, C. A. J., Savoy, L. A., & Darbre, P. D. (2012). Measurement of paraben concentrations in human breast tissue at serial locations across the breast from axilla to sternum. J Appl Toxicol, 32(3), 219–232.

23. Colliver, Victoria. "Study: BPA, Methylparaben Block Breast Cancer Drugs." SFGate. N.p., 13 Sept. 2011. Web. 26 Jan. 2015. <http://www.sfgate.com/news/article/Study-BPA-methylparaben-block-breast-cancer-2310172.php#photo-1818246>.

24. Environmental Working Group. Skin Deep. Parabens. Available online: http://www.cosmeticsdatabase.com/ingredient.php?ingred06=704450&refurl=%2Fproduct.php%3Fprod_id%3D17311%26. Accessed December 9, 2008.

25. Environmental Working Group. Skin Deep. Methylparaben. Available online: Environmental Working Group. Skin Deep. Parabens. Available online: http://www.cosmeticsdatabase.com/ingredient.php?ingred06=704450&refurl=%2Fproduct.php%3Fprod_id%3D17311%26. Accessed December 9, 2008.

26. Environmental Working Group. Skin Deep. Butylparaben. Available online: http://www.cosmeticsdatabase.com/ingredient.php?ingred06=700868. Accessed December 9, 2008.

27. Environmental Working Group. Skin Deep. Propylparaben. Available online: http://www.cosmeticsdatabase.com/ingredient.php?ingred06=705335. Accessed December 9, 2008.

28. Ishiwatari S, Suzuki T, Hitomi T, Yoshino T, Matsukuma S, Tsuji T. (2006). Effects of methyl paraben on skin keratinocytes. Journal of Applied Toxicology 27:1-9.)

29. "Butylated Hydroxyanisole CAS No. 25013-16-5." Report on Carcinogens. National Toxicology Program/ Department of Health and Human Services, n.d. Web. 26 Jan. 2015. <http://ntp.niehs.nih.gov/ntp/roc/content/profiles/butylatedhydroxyanisole.pdf#search=butylated%20hydroxyanisole>.

FOOD

1. Wells, Hodan Farrah., and Jean C. Buzby. *Dietary Assessment of Major Trends in U.S. Food Consumption, 1970-2005*. Washington, D.C.: USDA Economic Research Service, 2008. *Economic Research Service*. USDA, Mar. 2008. Web. 28 Jan. 2015. <http://www.ers.usda.gov/media/210677/ eib33_reportsummary_1_.pdf>.

2. Gunnars, Kris. "11 Graphs That Show Everything That Is Wrong With The Modern Diet." Authority Nutrition. N.p., 11 Feb. 2014. Web. 28 Jan. 2015. <http://authoritynutrition.com/ 11-graphs-that-show-what-is-wrong-with-modern-diet/>.

3. Taubes, Gary. "Is Sugar Toxic?" The New York Times. The New York Times, 16 Apr. 2011. Web. 28 Jan. 2015. <http:// www.nytimes.com/2011/04/17/magazine/mag-17Sugar-t.html? pagewanted=3&_r=1>.

4. "U.S. Food and Drug Administration." FDA Targets Trans Fat in Processed Foods. FDA7, 7 Nov. 2013. Web. 28 Jan. 2015. <http://www.fda.gov/ForConsumers/ConsumerUpdates/ ucm372915.htm>.

5. "What Are Hydrogenated Fats?" What Are Hydrogenated Fats? George Mateljan Foundation, n.d. Web. 26 Jan. 2015. <http:// www.whfoods.com/genpage.php?tname=george&dbid=10>.

6. Simopoulos, A.p. "The Importance of the Ratio of Omega-6/ omega-3 Essential Fatty Acids." Biomedicine & Pharmacotherapy 56.8 (2002): 365-79. Web.

7. Hemmelgarn, Melinda. "Fatty Acid Flip-Flop - Address Dietary Imbalance by Boosting Omega-3s, Decreasing Omega-6s." Today's Dietitian, Apr. 2011. Web. 28 Jan. 2015. <http:// www.todaysdietitian.com/newarchives/040511p48.shtml>.

8. Gonzalez, Acevedo, Sierra Hernandez, Martinez Salazar, PB Mandeville, Castillo Valadez, Mendoza De La Cruz, and Suarez Algara. "Effect of Omega 3 Fatty Acids on Body Female Obese Composition." Archives of Latin American Nutrition (2013): 224-31. Print.

9. "A Brief History of Olestra." A Brief History of Olestra. Center for Science in the Public Interest, n.d. Web. 28 Jan. 2015. <http://www.cspinet.org/olestra/history.html>.

10. Howard BV, Van Horn L, Hsia J, et al. Low-Fat Dietary Pattern and Risk of Cardiovascular Disease: The Women's Health Initiative Randomized Controlled Dietary Modification Trial. JAMA. 2006;295(6):655-666. doi:10.1001/jama.295.6.655.

11. Beresford, S. A. A. "Low-Fat Dietary Pattern and Risk of Colorectal Cancer: The Women's Health Initiative Randomized Controlled Dietary Modification Trial." JAMA: The Journal of the American Medical Association 295.6 (2006): 643-54. Web.

12. "Research Sheds Light on Gluten Issues." Research Sheds Light on Gluten Issues. Whole Grains Council, 25 Jan. 2012. Web. 28 Jan. 2015. <http://wholegrainscouncil.org/newsroom/blog/2012/01/research-sheds-light-on-gluten-issues>.

13. Mercola, Dr. "Is Something Wrong with Our Modern Diet?" Mercola.com. 24, 24 Feb. 2014. Web. 28 Jan. 2015. <http://articles.mercola.com/sites/articles/archive/2014/02/24/modern-diet.aspx>.

14. Held, Lisa E. "Are You Eating Frankenwheat?" Prevention. N.p., Nov. 2012. Web. 28 Jan. 2015. <http://www.prevention.com/food/healthy-eating-tips/why-modern-wheat-considered-frankenwheat>.

15. McAdams, Molly. "Are Eggs a Protein, Carbohydrate or Lipid?" Healthy Eating. SF Gate, n.d. Web. 28 Jan. 2015. <http://healthyeating.sfgate.com/eggs-protein-carbohydrate-lipid-1238.html>.

16. Wright, Carolanne. "Searching for a Good Egg: Which Type Is Best - Organic, Free-range, Pastured or Cage-free?" NaturalNews. Natural Health News & Self Reliance, 29 Jan. 2014. Web. 28 Jan. 2015. <http://www.naturalnews.com/043689_eggs_cage-free_organic_food.html>.

17. Servan-Schreiber, David. Anti Cancer: A New Way of Life. Melbourne, Australia: Scribe, 2008. Print.

18. Jampolis, Melina. "Is Farm-Raised Salmon As Healthy As Wise?" CNN. Cable News Network, 8 Jan. 2010. Web. 28 Jan. 2015. <http://www.cnn.com/2010/HEALTH/expert.q.a/01/08/salmon.fresh.farmed.jampolis/index.html>

19. Weiss, Kenneth. "Report Cites Health Risks of Farm-Raised Salmon." Los Angeles Times. Los Angeles Times, 09 Jan. 2004. Web. 28 Jan. 2015. <http://articles.latimes.com/2004/jan/09/local/me-salmon9>.

20. Huff, Ethan. "Unraveling Food Industry Lies - Your Salmon and Meat Are Artificially Dyed to Look More Appealing." NaturalNews. N.p., 10 Sept. 2012. Web. 28 Jan. 2015. <http://www.naturalnews.com/037136_food_industry_salmon_artificial_colors.html>.

21. Anderson, Stewart. Salmon Color and the Consumer (n.d.): n. pag. Oregonstate.edu. IIFET 2000 Proceedings. Web. 28 Jan. 2015. <http://oregonstate.edu/dept/IIFET/2000/papers/andersons.pdf>.

22. Roth, Alex. "The Salmon Struggle: A Fish by Any Other Color Is Just Not Natural." Seattlepi.com. N.p., 22 May 2003. Web. 28 Jan. 2015. <http://www.seattlepi.com/news/article/The-salmon-struggle-A-fish-by-any-other-color-is-1115339.php>.

23. Bottemiller, Helena. "Dispute Over Drug in Feed Limiting US Meat Exports - Food and Environment Reporting Network." Food and Environment Reporting Network. N.p., 24 Jan. 2012. Web. 28 Jan. 2015. <http://thefern.org/2012/01/dispute-over-drug-in-feed-limiting-u-s-meat-exports/>.

24. Yoquinto, Luke. "The Truth About Potassium Bromate." LiveScience. TechMedia Network, 16 Mar. 2012. Web. 28 Jan. 2015. <http://www.livescience.com/36206-truth-potassium-bromate-food-additive.html>.

25. Steve Kilburn, Tanya Moore, Gail Nelson, Barbara Roop, Ralph Slade, Adam Swank, William Ward, and Anthony Deangelo. "Molecular Biomarkers of Oxidative Stress Associated with Bromate Carcinogenicity." Toxicology 221.2-3 (2006): 158-65. Web. 28 Jan. 2015.

26. "CSPI Urges FDA to Ban Artificial Food Dyes Linked to Behavior Problems ~ Newsroom ~ News from CSPI ~ Center for Science in the Public Interest.", n.d. Web. 28 Jan. 2015. <http://www.cspinet.org/new/200806022.html>.

27. Stockman, J.a. "Food Additives and Hyperactive Behaviour in 3-year-old and 8/9-year-old Children in the Community: A Randomised, Double-blinded, Placebo-controlled Trial." Yearbook of Pediatrics 2009 (2009): 94-95. Web. 28 Jan. 2015.

28. Warner, Melanie. "FDA Hears From Critics on Artificial Food Dyes. Next Step: Ignore Them." CBSNews. CBS Interactive, 31 Mar. 2011. Web. 28 Jan. 2015. <http://www.cbsnews.com/news/fda-hears-from-critics-on-artificial-food-dyes-next-step-ignore-them/>.

29. "ECFR — Code of Federal Regulations." ECFR — Code of Federal Regulations. N.p., n.d. Web. 28 Jan. 2015. <http://www.ecfr.gov/cgi-bin/text-idx?c=ecfr&sid=3f6c9146ba54b1b84f17046e27197926&tpl=%2Fecfrbrowse%2FTitle21%2F21cfr74_main_02.tpl>

30. "Food Colouring | Food Processing." Encyclopedia Britannica Online. Encyclopedia Britannica, n.d. Web. 28 Jan. 2015. <http://www.britannica.com/EBchecked/topic/212658/food-colouring>.

31. Mercola, Joseph. "U.S. Foods Full of Banned Ingredients." Mercola.com. N.p., 27 Feb. 2013. Web. 27 Jan. 2015. <http://articles.mercola.com/sites/articles/archive/2013/02/27/us-food-products.aspx>.

32. Zeratsky, Katherine. "Nutrition and Healthy Eating." Brominated Vegetable Oil: Why Is BVO in My Drink? Mayo Clinic, 5 Apr. 2014. Web. 28 Jan. 2015. <http://www.mayoclinic.org/healthy-living/nutrition-and-healthy-eating/expert-answers/bvo/faq-20058236>.

33. "Recombinant Bovine Growth Hormone." Recombinant Bovine Growth Hormone. American Cancer Society, n.d. Web. 25 Jan. 2015. <http://www.cancer.org/cancer/cancercauses/

othercarcinogens/athome/recombinant-bovine-growth-hormone>.

34. "RbGH Milk Ruled "compositionally Different" by Ohio Court". GM Watch, n.d. Web. 28 Jan. 2015. <http://www.gmwatch.org/latest-listing/1-news-items/12566-rbgh-milk-ruled-qcompositionally-differentq-by-ohio-court>.

35. Haiken, Melanie. "Latest Food Scare: What Is The 'Yoga Mat' Chemical - And Why Is It In Your Food?" Forbes. Forbes Magazine, 27 Feb. 2014. Web. 28 Jan. 2015. <http://www.forbes.com/sites/melaniehaiken/2014/02/27/what-is-the-yoga-mat-chemical-and-why-is-it-in-your-food/>.

36. Cary, R., S. Dobson, and E. Ball. Azodicarbonamide. Geneva: World Health Organization, 1999. World Health Organization. World Health Organization, 1999. Web. 28 Jan. 2015. <http://www.who.int/ipcs/publications/cicad/en/cicad16.pdf>.

37. Yoquinto, Luke. "The Truth About Food Additive BHA." LiveScience. TechMedia Network, 01 June 2012. Web. 28 Jan. 2015. <http://www.livescience.com/36424-food-additive-bha-butylated-hydroxyanisole.html>.

38. Zerbe, Leah. "The Natural Ingredient You Should Ban From Your Diet." Prevention. N.p., n.d. Web. 28 Jan. 2015. <http://www.prevention.com/food/healthy-eating-tips/carrageenan-natural-ingredient-you-should-ban-your-diet>.

39. "Press Release." Centers for Disease Control and Prevention. Centers for Disease Control and Prevention, 16 Sept. 2013. Web. 27 Jan. 2015. <http://www.cdc.gov/media/releases/2013/p0916-untreatable.html>.

40. Bottemiller, Helena. "Most U.S. Antibiotics Go to Animal Agriculture." Food Safety News. N.p., 24 Feb. 2011. Web. 28 Jan. 2015. <http://www.foodsafetynews.com/2011/02/fda-confirms-80-percent-of-antibiotics-used-in-animal-ag/#.VGVNrvnF-So>.

41. Kilham, Chris. "Are Superbugs Linked to the Meat You Eat?" Fox News. FOX News Network, 14 Mar. 2013. Web. 28 Jan.

2015. <http://www.foxnews.com/health/2013/03/14/are-superbugs-linked-to-meat-eat/>.

42. Carpenter, Kenneth. "Journal of Nutrition." The Journal of Nutrition. The American Society for Nutritional Services, 17 Feb. 2000. Web. 28 Jan. 2015. <http://jn.nutrition.org/content/130/6/1521.full>.

43. Kennedy, Pagan. "The Fat Drug." The New York Times. The New York Times, 08 Mar. 2014. Web. 28 Jan. 2015. <http://www.nytimes.com/2014/03/09/opinion/sunday/the-fat-drug.html?_r=0>.

44. Robinson, Allan. "Food Additives: What Is Sodium Phosphate?" LIVESTRONG.COM. LIVESTRONG.COM, 06 Sept. 2013. Web. 28 Jan. 2015. <http://www.livestrong.com/article/40858-sodium-phosphate-label/>.

45. Greger, Michael. "Phosphate Additives in Chicken Banned Elsewhere." NutritionFacts.org. N.p., 16 Oct. 2014. Web. 28 Jan. 2015. <http://nutritionfacts.org/2014/10/16/phosphate-additives-in-chicken-banned-elsewhere/>.

46. Ritz, Eberhard et al. "Phosphate Additives in Food—a Health Risk." Deutsches Ärzteblatt International 109.4 (2012): 49–55. PMC. Web. 28 Jan. 2015.

47. Calvo, Mona S., and Katherine L. Tucker. "Is Phosphorus Intake That Exceeds Dietary Requirements a Risk Factor in Bone Health?" Annals of the New York Academy of Sciences 1301.1 (2013): 29-35. Web.

48. "Monsanto: A History." GM Watch, 6 Feb. 2009. Web. 28 Jan. 2015. <http://gmwatch.org/gm-firms/10595-monsanto-a-history>.

49. King, Joe, MS. "Side Effects of Saccharin Sodium." LIVESTRONG.COM. LIVESTRONG.COM, 14 June 2011. Web. 28 Jan. 2015. <http://www.livestrong.com/article/470503-side-effects-of-saccharin-sodium/>.

50. "Metroactive Features." Metroactive Features | Monsanto Company. Metro, Silicon Valley's Weekly Newspaper., 11 May

2000. Web. 28 Jan. 2015. <http://www.metroactive.com/papers/metro/05.11.00/cover/gen-food2-0019.html>.

51. "Polystyrene Fast Facts." (n.d.): n. pag. The Way To Go. Harvard.edu, 2008. Web. 28 Jan. 2015. <http://isites.harvard.edu/fs/docs/icb.topic967858.files/PolystyreneFactSheets.pdf>.

52. Lah, Katrina, and Maria Mergel. "2,4,5-T." Toxepedia. N.p., 6 Apr. 2011. Web. 29 Jan. 2015. <http%3A%2F%2Fwww.toxipedia.org%2Fdisplay%2Ftoxiped ia%2F2%252C4%252C5-T>.

53. "DDT." EPA. Environmental Protection Agency, n.d. Web. 27 Jan. 2015. <http://www.epa.gov/pbt/pubs/ddt.htm>.

54. Gillam, Carey. "Heavy Use of Herbicide Roundup Linked to Health Dangers-U.S. Study." Reuters. Thomson Reuters, 25 Apr. 2013. Web. 29 Jan. 2015. <http://www.reuters.com/article/2013/04/25/roundup-health-study-idUSL2N0DC22F20130425>.

55. Grunwald, Michael. "Monsanto Hid Decades Of Pollution." Common Dreams. N.p., 1 Jan. 2002. Web. 29 Jan. 2015. <http://www.commondreams.org/headlines02/0101-02.htm>.

56. Gurian-Sherman, Doug. "Failure to Yield." (n.d.): n. pag. Union of Concerned Scientists USA. Apr. 2009. Web. 29 Jan. 2015. <http://www.ucsusa.org/sites/default/files/legacy/assets/documents/food_and_agriculture/failure-to-yield.pdf>.

57. "Genetically Modified Foods." Position Paper:: The American Academy of Environmental Medicine (AAEM). American Academy of Environmental Medicine, n.d. Web. 29 Jan. 2015. <http://www.aaemonline.org/gmopost.html>.

58. "Institute for Responsible Technology." 10 Reasons to Avoid GMOs. Institute for Responsible Technology, n.d. Web. 28 Jan. 2015. <http://responsibletechnology.org/10-Reasons-to-Avoid-GMOs>.

59. Mellon, Margaret, and Jane Rissler. "Not Gone to Seed." Science 286.5447 (1999): 2041k-041. Union of Concerned Scientists USA. 2009. Web. 29 Jan. 2015. <http://

www.ucsusa.org/sites/default/files/legacy/assets/documents/
food_and_agriculture/seedreport_fullreport.pdf>.

60. Hoover, Angela. "Leave a Comment." Poor Gut Health And Autism Linked Through GMOs (Genetically Modified Organisms). Health and Wellness Magazine, 1 Apr. 2013. Web. 29 Jan. 2015. <http://healthandwellnessmagazine.net/content/features/poor-gut-health-and-autism-linked-through-gmos-genetically-modified-organisms/>.

61. Schnabl, Bernd. "Linking Intestinal Homeostasis and Liver Disease." Current Opinion in Gastroenterology 29.3 (2013): 264-70. Web.

62. Saggioro, A. "Leaky Gut, Microbiota, and Cancer: An Incoming Hypothesis." Journal of Clinical Gastroenterology 48 (2014): 62-66. Web.

63. Rogler, G., and G. Rosana. "The Heart and the Gut." European Heart Journal 35.7 (2014): 426-430. Print.

64. Roberts, James, and Catherine Karr. "Pesticide Exposure in Children." Pediatrics. American Academy of Pediatrics, n.d. Web. 29 Jan. 2015. <http://m.pediatrics.aappublications.org/content/130/6/e1757.full>.

65. "USDA Quietly Approves More GE Corn, Considering Key Agent Orange Ingredient." 10 Jan. 2012. Web. 29 Jan. 2015. <http://www.sustainablebusiness.com/index.cfm/go/news.display/id/23302>.

66. McIntyre, Beverly, Et Al. "Agriculture at a Crossroads." (n.d.): n. pag. International Assessment of Agricultural Knowledge, Science and Technology for Development. Web. 29 Jan. 2015. <http://www.unep.org/dewa/agassessment/reports/IAASTD/EN/Agriculture%20at%20a%20Crossroads_Global%20Report%20(English).pdf>.

67. Robbins, Ocean. "Did Monsanto Trick California Voters?" The Huffington Post. TheHuffingtonPost.com, 8 Jan. 2013. Web. 29 Jan. 2015. <http://www.huffingtonpost.com/ocean-robbins/monsanto-prop-37_b_2088934.html>.

68. "USDA ERS - Organic Agriculture." USDA ERS - Organic Agriculture. United States Department of Agriculture, n.d. Web. 29 Jan. 2015. <http://www.ers.usda.gov/topics/natural-resources-environment/organic-agriculture.aspx>.

69. "Eating Healthy with Cruciferous Vegetables." Eating Healthy with Cruciferous Vegetables. George Mateljan Foundationan Foundation, n.d. Web. 29 Jan. 2015. <http://www.whfoods.com/genpage.php?tname=btnews&dbid=126>.

70. Krause, Marie V., L. Kathleen. Mahan, and Sylvia Escott-Stump. Food, Nutrition, and Diet Therapy. Philadelphia: Saunders, 1996. Print.

71. Losso, J., R. Bansode, A. Trappeyii, H. Bawadi, and R. Truax. "In Vitro Anti-proliferative Activities of Ellagic Acid." The Journal of Nutritional Biochemistry 15.11 (2004): 672-78. Web.

72. Li, TM, GW Chen, CC Su, JG Lin, CC Yeh, KC Cheng, and JG Chung. "Ellagic Acid Induced P53/p21 Expression, G1 Arrest and Apoptosis in Human Bladder Cancer T24 Cells." Anticancer Research 25.2A (2005): 971-79. Web. 29 Jan. 2015.

73. Malar DS, Devi KP . "Dietary polyphenols for treatment of Alzheimer's disease--future research and development." Curr Pharm Biotechnol. 2014;15(4):330-42.

74. "Flavonoids." Flavonoids. George Mateljan Foundationan Foundation, n.d. Web. 29 Jan. 2015. <http://www.whfoods.com/genpage.php?tname=nutrient&dbid=119>.

75. "Evaluation of the effects of swainsonine, captopril, tangeretin and nobiletin on the biological behaviour of brain tumour cells in vitro." Neuropathol Appl Neurobiol. 2001 Feb;27(1):29-39. Rooprai HK1, Kandanearatchi A, Maidment SL, Christidou M, Trillo-Pazos G, Dexter DT, Rucklidge GJ, Widmer W, Pilkington GJ.) and (Cancer Chemother Pharmacol. 2014 Nov 28. [Epub ahead of print]

76. Periyasamy, K., K. Baskaran, A. Illakkia, K. Vanitha, S. Selvaraj, and D. Sakthisekaran. "Antitumor Efficacy of Tangeretin by Targeting the Oxidative Stress Mediated on 7,12-

dimethylbenz(a) Anthracene-induced Proliferative Breast Cancer in Sprague-Dawley Rats." *Cancer Chemotherapy and Pharmacology* 75.2 (2015): 263-72. Web. 29 Jan. 2015.

77. "Chemopreventive and therapeutic potential of "naringenin," a flavanone present in citrus fruits." Mir IA1, Tiku AB Nutr Cancer. 2015 Jan;67(1):27-42. doi: 10.1080/01635581.2015.976320. Epub 2014 Dec 16.

78. "Combination of Ethanolic Extract of Citrus aurantifolia Peels with Doxorubicin Modulate Cell Cycle and Increase Apoptosis Induction on MCF-7 Cells." Adina AB1, Goenadi FA1, Handoko FF1, Nawangsari DA1, Hermawan A1, Jenie RI1, Meiyanto E1 Iran J Pharm Res. 2014 Summer;13(3):919-26.

79. "Effects of the Olive-Derived Polyphenol Oleuropein on Human Health." Barbaro, Barbara et al. Ed. Segura-Carretero Antonio. International Journal of Molecular Sciences 15.10 (2014): 18508–18524. PMC. Web. 5 Jan. 2015.

80. Menendez JA1, Vazquez-Martin A, Oliveras-Ferraros C, Garcia-Villalba R, Carrasco-Pancorbo A, Fernandez-Gutierrez A, Segura-Carretero A "Analyzing effects of extra-virgin olive oil polyphenols on breast cancer-associated fatty acid synthase protein expression using reverse-phase protein microarrays."(Int J Mol Med. 2008 Oct;22(4):433-9..

81. Ng ML, Yap AT. Inhibition of human colon carcinoma development by lentinan from shiitake mushrooms (Lentinus edodes). J Altern Complement Med 2002;8(5):581-589.

82. Taggart, Rebecca. "The Wonderful World of Alliums." The Wonderful World of Alliums. The Fruit Guys Magazine, May 2009. Web. 29 Jan. 2015. <http://fruitguys.com/almanac/2012/05/09/the-wonderful-world-of-alliums>.

83. "Home Page." NYU Langone Medical Center. N.p., n.d. Web. 28 Jan. 2015. <http://www.med.nyu.edu/content?ChunkIID=21729>.

84. Garland, Cedric F. et al. "The Role of Vitamin D in Cancer Prevention." American Journal of Public Health 96.2 (2006): 252–261. PMC. Web. 5 Jan. 2015.

85. Sacks, Dr. Frank. "Ask the Expert: Omega-3 Fatty Acids." The Nutrition Source. Harvard, n.d. Web. 27 Jan. 2015. <http://www.hsph.harvard.edu/nutritionsource/omega-3/>.

86. "Search Results." Foods Highest in Total Omega-3 Fatty Acids. Self, n.d. Web. 29 Jan. 2015. <http://nutritiondata.self.com/foods-000140000000000000000.html>.

87. Smith, Michael, and Laura Martin. "Probiotics and Prebiotics: Ask the Nutritionist on WebMD." WebMD. WebMD, n.d. Web. 29 Jan. 2015. <http://www.webmd.com/vitamins-and-supplements/nutrition-vitamins-11/probiotics>.

88. "Role Of Probiotics And Functional Foods In Health: Gut Immune Stimulation By Two Probiotic Strains And A Potential Probiotic Yoghurt." Galdeano CM, Nuñez IN, Carmuega E, de LeBlanc AD, Perdigón G1. (Endocr Metab Immune Disord Drug Targets. 2014 Dec 16. [Epub ahead of print]

89. "What Are Some of the Best Food Sources for Probiotics and Prebiotics?" What Are Some of the Best Food Sources for Probiotics and Prebiotics? George Mateljan Foundationan Foundation, n.d. Web. 29 Jan. 2015. <http://whfoods.org/genpage.php?tname=dailytip&dbid=113>.

90. Mercola, Dr. "Enzymes: Food That Slow Nearly Every Inflammatory Disease." Mercola.com. N.p., 21 Aug. 2011. Web. 29 Jan. 2015. <http://articles.mercola.com/sites/articles/archive/2011/08/21/enzymes-special-report.aspx>.

91. Carter, Andrea. "Curry Compound Fights Cancer in the Clinic." (n.d.): n. pag. JNCI. Oxford Journals. Web. 29 Jan. 2015. <http://jnci.oxfordjournals.org/content/100/9/616.full.pdf>.

92. "Tea and Cancer Prevention." National Cancer Institute. National Institutes of Health, n.d. Web. 29 Jan. 2015. <http://www.cancer.gov/cancertopics/factsheet/prevention/tea>.

93. Essential Oils Desk Reference. U.S.A.: Life Science Pub., 2011. Print.

94. Chaudhary, S., M. Siddiqui, M. Athar, and M. S. Alam. "D-Limonene Modulates Inflammation, Oxidative Stress and Ras-

ERK Pathway to Inhibit Murine Skin Tumorigenesis." Human & Experimental Toxicology 31.8 (2012): 798-811. Web.

95. Hyman, MD Mark. "Glutathione: The Mother of All Antioxidants." The Huffington Post. TheHuffingtonPost.com, n.d. Web. 29 Jan. 2015. <http://www.huffingtonpost.com/dr-mark-hyman/glutathione-the-mother-of_b_530494.html>.

96. Welch, Ailsa, Alex Macgregor, Amy Jennings, Sue Fairweather-Tait, Tim Spector, and Aedín Cassidy. "Habitual Flavonoid Intakes Are Positively Associated with Bone Mineral Density in Women." Journal of Bone and Mineral Research 27.9 (2012): 1872-1878. Web.

97. Gao, X., A. Cassidy, MA Schwarzschild, EB Rimm, and A. Acherio. "Habitual Intake of Dietary Flavonoids and Risk of Parkinson Disease." Habitual Intake of Dietary Flavonoids and Risk of Parkinson Disease. Neurology, 4 Apr. 2012. Web. 29 Jan. 2015. <http://www.neurology.org/content/early/2012/04/04/WNL.0b013e31824f7fc4>.

98. "Lutein & Zeaxanthin." Lutein & Zeaxanthin. American Optometric Association, n.d. Web. 29 Jan. 2015. <http://www.aoa.org/patients-and-public/caring-for-your-vision/diet-and-nutrition/lutein>.

99. Hubbard, Sylvia. "7 Cancer-Fighting Food Combos." NewsmaxHealth. N.p., 02 May 2014. Web. 29 Jan. 2015. <http://www.newsmaxhealth.com/Headline/food-synergy-cancer-protection/2014/05/01/id/569040/>.

100. Magee, MPH, RDWebMD Weight Loss Clinic-Feature, Elaine. "Top 10 Food Synergy Super Foods." WebMD. WebMD, n.d. Web. 29 Jan. 2015. <http://www.webmd.com/food-recipes/features/top-10-food-synergy-super-foods>.

101. Andrew J. McDermott, ENS, MC, USN; Mark B. Stephens, MD, CAPT, MC, USN April 2010 Family Medicine Cost of Eating: Whole Foods Versus Convenience Foods in a Low-income Model.

102. "EWG's 2014 Shopper's Guide to Pesticides in Produce™." EWG's 2014 Shopper's Guide to Pesticides in Produce™.

Environmental Working Group, 2014. Web. 27 Jan. 2015. <http://www.ewg.org/foodnews/summary.php>.

103. Yan, Holly. "Jurors Give $289 Million to a Man They Say Got Cancer from Monsanto's Roundup Weedkiller." *CNN*, Cable News Network, 12 Aug. 2018, www.cnn.com/2018/08/10/health/monsanto-johnson-trial-verdict/index.html

NATURAL HEALTH

1. "Cancer." WHO. World Health Organization, Nov. 2014. Web. 27 Jan. 2015. <http://www.who.int/mediacentre/factsheets/fs297/en/>.

2. "FAERS Reporting by Patient Outcomes by Year." FAERS Reporting by Patient Outcomes by Year. US Food and Drug Administration, 31 Dec. 2013. Web. 30 Jan. 2015. <http://www.fda.gov/Drugs/GuidanceComplianceRegulatoryInformation/Surveillance/AdverseDrugEffects/ucm070461.htm>.

3. Fassa, Paul. "Beware of The #1 Cause of Acute Liver Damage." REALfarmacy.com. N.p., 14 May 2014. Web. 30 Jan. 2015. <http://www.realfarmacy.com/beware-of-the-1-cause-of-acute-liver-damage/>.

4. Bollinger, Ty. The Truth About Cancer - The Quest for the Cures Continues. Complete 11 Episode Transcripts. USA: TTAC , LLC, 2014. Print.

5. Duffy, Thomas P., MD. "The Flexner Report - 100 Years Later." Yale Journal of Biology and Medicine 84 (2011): 269-276. Print.

6. Servan-Schreiber, David. Anticancer: A New Way of Life. New York: Viking, 2008. Print.

7. "Lipitor Side Effects in Detail - Drugs.com." Lipitor Side Effects in Detail - Drugs.com. Drugs.com, n.d. Web. 30 Jan. 2015. <http://www.drugs.com/sfx/lipitor-side-effects.html>.

8. Essential Oils Desk Reference. U.S.A.: Life Science Pub., 2011. Print.

9. Schnaubelt, Kurt. The Healing Intelligence of Essential Oils: The Science of Advanced Aromatherapy. Rochester, VT: Healing Arts, 2011. Print.

10. Akihisa, Toshihiro, Keiichi Tabata, Norihiro Banno, Harukuni Tokuda, Reiko Nishihara, Yuji Nakamura, Yumiko Kimura, Ken Yasukawa, and Takashi Suzuki. "Cancer Chemopreventive Effects and Cytotoxic Activities of the Triterpene Acids from the Resin of Boswellia Carteri." Biological & Pharmaceutical Bulletin 29.9 (2006): 1976-1979. Web.

11. Wang, R., Y. Wang, Z. Gao, and X. Qu. "The Comparative Study of Acetyl-11-keto-beta-boswellic Acid (AKBA) and Aspirin in the Prevention of Intestinal Adenomatous Polyposis in APC(Min/+) Mice." Drug Discoveries and Therapeutics 8.1 (2014): 25-32. Web.

12. Ni, Xiao, Mahmoud M. Suhail, Qing Yang, Amy Cao, Kar-Ming Fung, Russell G. Postier, Cole Woolley, Gary Young, Jingzhe Zhang, and Hsueh-Kung Lin. "Frankincense Essential Oil Prepared from Hydrodistillation of Boswellia Sacra Gum Resins Induces Human Pancreatic Cancer Cell Death in Cultures and in a Xenograft Murine Model." BMC Complementary and Alternative Medicine 12.1 (2012): 253. Web.

13. Ni, Xiao, Mahmoud M. Suhail, Qing Yang, Amy Cao, Kar-Ming Fung, Russell G. Postier, Cole Woolley, Gary Young, Jingzhe Zhang, and Hsueh-Kung Lin. "Frankincense Essential Oil Prepared from Hydrodistillation of Boswellia Sacra Gum Resins Induces Human Pancreatic Cancer Cell Death in Cultures and in a Xenograft Murine Model." BMC Complementary and Alternative Medicine 12.1 (2012): 253. Web.

14. Frank, Mark, Qing Yang, Jeanette Osban, Joseph T. Azzarello, Marcia R. Saban, Ricardo Saban, Richard A. Ashley, Jan C. Welter, Kar-Ming Fung, and Hsueh-Kung Lin. "Frankincense Oil Derived from Boswellia Carteri Induces Tumor Cell

Specific Cytotoxicity." BMC Complementary and Alternative Medicine 9.1 (2009): 6. Web.

15. Suhail, Mahmoud M., Weijuan Wu, Amy Cao, Fadee G. Mondalek, Kar-Ming Fung, Pin-Tsen Shih, Yu-Ting Fang, Cole Woolley, Gary Young, and Hsueh-Kung Lin. "Boswellia Sacra Essential Oil Induces Tumor Cell-specific Apoptosis and Suppresses Tumor Aggressiveness in Cultured Human Breast Cancer Cells." BMC Complementary and Alternative Medicine 11.1 (2011): 129. Web.

16. Fung KM, Suhail MM, McClendon B, Woolley CL, Young DG, Lin HK. Management of basal cell carcinoma of the skin using frankincense (Boswellia sacra) essential oil: A case report. OA Alternative Medicine 2013 Jun 01;1(2):14.

17. "NIH Budget - About NIH - National Institutes of Health (NIH)." U.S National Library of Medicine. U.S. National Library of Medicine, n.d. Web. 30 Jan. 2015. <http://www.nih.gov/about/budget.htm>.

18. Dahl, Julie. "REO Foundation." (n.d.): n. pag. Research Essential Oils. REO Foundation. Web. 30 Jan. 2015. <http://www.reo-foundation.org/wp-content/uploads/2014/06/REO-letter-for-donations-LONG-signed.pdf>.

Acknowledgements

My girls: Maggie, Sarah Jayne, and Genevieve - You are the reason I get up and do what I do each day. Because of you, my passion for and my commitment to living as healthily as possible will never wane. I love each of you to the moon and back!

My David- There aren't enough words to cover all the ways I love you. I will be forever in awe and grateful for the way you love me unconditionally.

Mom and Dad - We couldn't have made it through the past two years without y'all! I love you both very much.

My sisters, Jennifer and Sally - Thank you for loving and supporting me from across the miles. I love and miss both of you so much!

Marjorie Williams - Thank you for raising a wonderful man who is the best husband and father a gal could ask for!

Louisa, Saint Louisa - Thank you for caring for my babies just like you do your own boys. You are a blessing to our family.

Ashley Farless - I thank my lucky stars for you, my sista from another mista. I never thought sitting together in the chemo room would be on our bucket list. I am happy you were there to hold my hand and make me laugh!

Kate West - You make me happy when skies are grey. Thank you for bringing your sunshine all the way to Texas! I thank God for you!

Crystal Burchfield - I thank you for always lending an ear and for encouraging me to write this book. You changed my life when you introduced me to Young Living!

Heather Walsh - Thank you for being there any time I needed a helping hang. You have cheered me on every step of the way.

Jeanne Batey - You make me laugh, which is my favorite thing in the whole wide world. Thank you for encouraging me to write and for keeping me giggling along the way.

Whitney McGinlay - Thank you for taking Sarah Jayne as your third child on so many occasions!

Betty Allen - I thank you for all of your sage and pertinent advice...you always know just what to say. I heart you, my MILS.

Carole Elledge - You are the best personal cancer guide! I'd have been totally lost without you.

Regina Austin - You made seeing "the gals" off super fun! Thank you for being a constant source of support and good advice.

Fawn Creamer, my birthday twin - I am so grateful that serendipity brought me such a fun and caring friend. Thank you for keeping me laughing throughout dark times!

My Local Team: Natalie, Wendy, Haley, Laini, Heather, JJ, Elizabeth, and Pam - Thank you for shuffling my kids around and feeding my family!

Ashley Williams, Anna Hudson, LeeAnn Collins, April Boswell, Lanis Marbut, Becky Cantrell, Deb Findley - Thank you for always reaching across the miles to check on me!

Pink Sisters, my online Breast Friends- Thank you for being there day or night to answer questions and offer love, support, and laughs!

God - couldn't have done it without you. (I probably should have listed You first...but I guess I saved the best for last.)

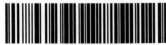

Made in the USA
Lexington, KY
16 October 2018